HEALTHY AND EASY RECIPE

DONNA WHITE

Copyright© 2019 by Donna White

All rights reserved. This book or any portion thereof my not be reproduced or used in any manner whatsoever without the express written permission of the publisher.

Table of Contents

Spicy Pork And Sweet Potato Stew 1

Spicy Sweet Shrimp With Pineapple Sa 5

Roasted Brussels Sprouts With Bacon 8

Baked Butter Garlic Shrimp 11

One-Pan Egg & Veg Brunch 14

Pasta With Salmon & Peas 17

Pappardelle Broad Bean Carbonara 19

Tomatoes Stuffed With Pesto Rice 22

Herb-And-Mustard Sirloin With Baked Potatoes .. 24

Chicken-And-Cheese Enchiladas 27

Pita Pizzas 30

Roasted Brussels Sprouts With Bacon 33

Cauliflower Toast With Avocado 36

One-Pot Paprika Cod And Chickpeas 39

Zucchini & Sausage Stovetop Casserole 41

Steak & Mushroom Stroganoff 44

Parmesan Chicken With Lemon Rice.................. 47

Grilled Salmon With Chorizo-Olive Sauce 50

Beef & Bacon Gnocchi Skillet.................. 53

Chili Dog Pizza 56

Chicken Tamale Bake 58

Ginger Halibut With Brussels Sprouts 61

One-Pot Spinach Beef Soup.................. 64

Bucatini With Sausage & Kale.................. 67

Bbq Hot Dog & Potato Packs 70

Grilled Chicken Chopped Salad.................. 72

Spicy Shrimp & Watermelon Kabobs 75

Pizza In A Bowl.................. 78

Cauliflower & Tofu Curry 80

Lemon-Garlic Pork Chops.................. 83

Apple & Sweet Potato Quinoa 85

Haddock With Lime-Cilantro Butter.................. 88

Hoisin Turkey Lettuce Wraps 90

Waffle-Iron Pizzas 92

Southern Pork & Rice... 94

Cheesy Chicken & Broccoli Orzo 97

Apple, White Cheddar & Arugula Tarts 99

Grilled Citrus Salmon.. 101

Zesty Grilled Chops.. 103

Caribbean Shrimp & Rice Bowl 105

Sausage-Stuffed Butternut Squash....................... 108

Spicy Chicken Nuggets 111

Scallops With Wilted Spinach 113

Mom's Spanish Rice 115

Easy Buffalo Chicken Dip 117

Better Than Fried Shrimp 119

Walnut-Crusted Salmon... 121

Grilled Honey-Lime Chicken 123

Honey Grilled Shrimp.. 125

Corn With Cilantro-Lime Butter........................... 127

Grilled Huli Huli Chicken..................................... 129

Grilled Vegetable Platter.. 132

Contest-Winning Grilled Mushrooms................. 135

30-Minute Chicken Noodle Soup 137

Grilled Fajitas 139

Grilled Potato Skins 142

Rice On The Grill 145

Balsamic-Glazed Beef Skewers 147

Hot Quick Banana Boats...................................... 149

Spinach And Mushroom Smothered Chicken 151

Mushroom Cheese Bread 154

Grilled Tilapia Piccata 156

Bruschetta From The Grill.................................... 159

Ultimate Grilled Pork Chops................................. 162

Blue Cheese & Bacon Stuffed Peppers 165

Summer Steak Kabobs 167

Grilled Potatoes With Bacon-Ranch Sauce 170

Flank Steak With Cilantro & Blue Cheese Butter 172

Grilled Jalapenos 175

Grilled Pork Tenderloins 177

Triple Tomato Flatbread 180

Italian Sausage And Provolone Skewers 183

Chicken Caprese Zoodle Bowls 185

Low Carb Pizza Chicken Skillet 187

Tequila Lime Chicken 190

Chicken And Cauliflower Skillet 193

Broiled Chicken Thighs With Artichokes And Garlic 196

Cumin Spiced Beef Wraps – Low Carb, Paleo 199

Lemon And Thyme Chicken Thighs 202

Grilled Chicken, Bacon & Radishes 206

Pan Seared Chicken Breast With Mustard Cream .. 209

Sauce (Low Carb, Gluten-Free) 209

Easy Pan Seared Lamb Chops With Mustard Cream Sauce 213

Greek Herbed Lamb 218

Perfect Bacon And Egg Cups 222

Roasted Brussels Sprouts With Bacon 224

Easy Turkey Chili Recipe 227

County Fair Cinnamon Donuts 230

Cookie Dough Recipe No Eggs 234

Almond Milk Ice Cream Recipe 236

Chewy Granola Bar Recipe 238

Blueberry Coconut Porridge 241

Blini Style Caviar Crepes 244

Pumpkin Macadamia Butter 247

Brie & Apple Crepes 249

Grandma's Honey Muffins 252

Taco Cracker 255

Lemon And Thyme Chicken Thighs 257

Plant Based Recipes 261

Vegetarian Tortilla Soup 261

Sweet Potato And Black Bean Tacos 266

Grilled Cauliflower Wedges 272

Roasted Balsamic Red Potatoes 274

Easy Homemade Chunky Applesauce 276

Mushroom & Broccoli Soup 281

Avocado Fruit Salad With Tangerine Vinaigrette . 284

Roasted Curried Chickpeas And Cauliflower 287

Chickpea Mint Tabbouleh 289

Creamy Cauliflower Pakora Soup 292

Spice Trade Beans & Bulgur 295

Garden Vegetable & Herb Soup 298

Meat Based Recipes 301

Meat Loaf Minia 301

Bacon-Topped Meat Loaf 304

Easy Asian Glazed Meatballs 306

Asian-Style Round Steak.................................. 309

Meat Loaf Dinner 312

Pressure Cooker Mushroom Pot Roast................ 314

Chewy Granola Bar Recipe..................................... 318

Blueberry Coconut Porridge 321

Blini Style Caviar Crepes 324

Chicken Caprese Zoodle Bowls 327

Low Carb Pizza Chicken Skillet............................. 330

Tequila Lime Chicken... 333

Chicken And Cauliflower Skillet............................ 336

Broiled Chicken Thighs With Artichokes And Garlic
.... 339

Key Lime Cheesecake Bars...................................... 342

Keto Peppermint Chocolate.................................... 345

Low Carb Lemon Cheesecake 348

Keto Chocolate Chip Cookies 352

Keto Peanut Butter Tagalong Bars......................... 355

- Keto Shortbread Cookies 359
- Keto Chocolate Mousse 363
- Keto Carrot Cake 365
- Flourless Keto Brownies 369
- Keto Pumpkin Spice Muffins With Almond Flour 372
- Keto Moulds Bars 376
- Baked Lobster Tails With Garlic Butter 380
- Summer Berry And Burrata Salad 383
- Chicken Caprese Zoodle Bowls 387
- Low Carb Pizza Chicken Skillet 390
- Greek Herbed Lamb 393
- Seared Tuna Steak 397
- Quick And Easy Recipe Easy 399
- Bok Choy Chicken Recipe 399
- Garlic Butter Steak Recipe 404
- Parmesan Garlic Bread Recipe 408
- Ginger Soy Bok Choy Recipe 411

Asian-Brined Pork Chops Recipe 414

Garlic Noodles Recipe 418

Roasted Asparagus With Garlic Recipe.................. 423

Baked Chicken And Potato Casserole Recipe.... 426

Italian Shrimp Pasta Recipe 430

Garlic Parmesan Roasted Carrots Recipe 434

Garlic Herb Grilled Salmon Recipe 438

Baked Chicken Wings Recipe 443

Sweet And Sour Pork Noodles Recipe 446

Crispy Baked Orange Chicken Wings Recipe 450

Pomelo Salad: Yam Som-O Recipe 455

One Pot Meatball Casserole Recipe 461

Thai Peanut Zucchini Noodles Recipe 465

Tandoori Chicken Recipe 469

Spam Fried Rice Recipe... 473

Kung Pao Shrimp Recipe 477

Creamy Thai Coconut Chicken Soup Recipe 482

Roasted Bok Choy...487

Black Pepper Shrimp Recipe 491

SPICY PORK AND SWEET POTATO STEW

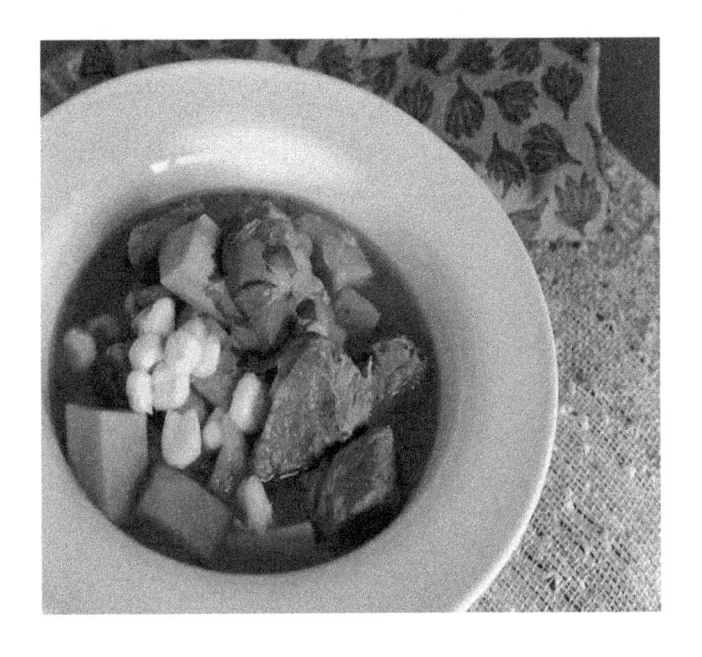

PREP: 10 MIN
COOK: 20 MIN
CARBS PER MEAL: 48g

Ingrgdients

1. 1 cup canned unsalted diced tomatoes

2. medium white onion, quartered

3. cloves garlic
4. 1/2 chipotle in adobo sauce, plus 1 tablespoon of the sauce
5. 2 tablespoons vegetable oil
6. 1 large pork tenderloin, trimmed and cut into 1-inch chunks (about 1 1/2 pounds)
7. Kosher salt and freshly ground black pepper
8. tablespoon chili powder
9. One 8-ounce sweet potato, peeled and cut into 1/2-inch chunks
10. 1cups low-sodium chicken broth
11. 1 tablespoon pickled jalapenos
12. 1 cup 2 percent Greek yogurt
13. 11/4 medium head red cabbage
14. 1 medium Haas avocado
15. 1 lime
16. 1/2 cup loosely packed fresh cilantro
17. Eight 6-inch corn tortillas, warmed

INSTRUCTIONS:

Puree the tomatoes, onions, garlic, chipotle and adobo sauce in a food processor until completely smooth.

Heat the oil in a large Dutch oven or pot over medium-high heat until nearly smoking. Add the pork in a single layer, season with 1 teaspoon salt and 1/2 teaspoon pepper and cook, undisturbed, until beginning to brown, about 2 minutes. Turn the pieces and cook until brown, about 1 minute more. Dust the meat with the chili powder, and add the tomato puree, sweet potatoes, chicken broth, 1/4 teaspoon salt and a few grinds of pepper. Bring to a boil, reduce the heat to medium, cover and gently simmer until the meat is cooked through and the potatoes are tender, about 15 minutes.

Meanwhile, prepare the toppings: Chop the jalapenos, and whisk together with the yogurt in a small bowl. Shred the cabbage, cut the avocado into chunks and cut the lime into wedges.

Ladle the stew into large, deep bowls. Top with the yogurt mixture, garnish with the cabbage, avocado, lime and cilantro and serve with the tortillas.

Spicy Sweet Shrimp with Pineapple Sa

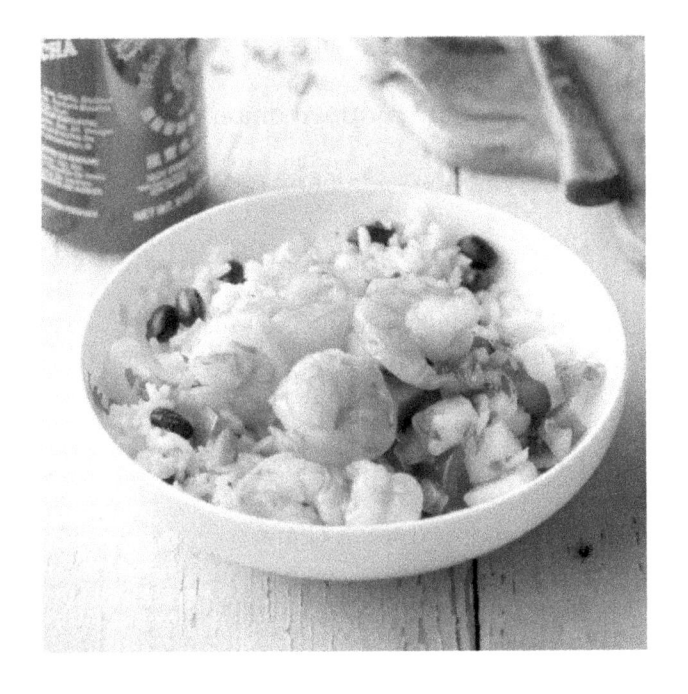

Prep:15 min
Cook:15min
Carbs per meal: 59g

INGREDIENTS:

1. 1-1/2 cups uncooked basmati rice

2. 3/4 cup canned black beans, rinsed and drained
3. 2 teaspoons canola oil
4. 1/2 cup finely chopped onion
5. 1-1/2 cups unsweetened pineapple juice
6. 1/4 cup packed brown sugar
7. 1 tablespoon Sriracha chili sauce
8. 3 cups cubed fresh pineapple
9. 1 medium sweet red pepper, diced
10. 1 cup chopped fresh cilantro
11. small red onion, finely chopped
12. tablespoons lime juice
13. 1/4 teaspoon salt
14. 1/4 teaspoon pepper
15. 1-1/2 pounds peeled and deveined shrimp (31-40 per pound)

INSTRUCTIONS:

- Cook rice according to package directions. Stir in beans; cover and keep warm.

- While rice cooks, heat oil in a large skillet over medium-high heat. Saute onion until tender, 3-4 minutes. Stir in pineapple juice, brown sugar and chili sauce; bring to a boil. Cook, uncovered, on high until liquid is reduced to 1/2 cup, 10-12 minutes.

- For salsa, toss pineapple with red pepper, cilantro, red onion, lime juice, salt and pepper.

- Once sauce has reduced, stir in shrimp and return just to a boil. Reduce heat; simmer, uncovered, until shrimp turns pink, 2-3 minutes. Serve with rice mixture and salsa.

ROASTED BRUSSELS SPROUTS WITH BACON

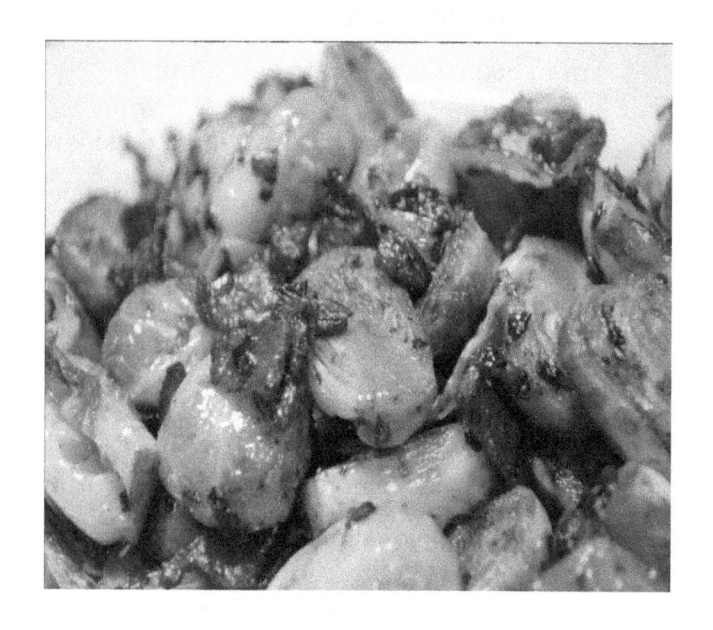

Prep time: 5 mins
Cook time: 30 mins
Carbs per meal: 27g

Ingredients

1. Lb brussels sprouts
2. tbsp olive oil 8 strips bacon   salt pepper

Instructions

- Preheat the oven to 375°F and cut the ends off of each brussels sprout, it's too tough. Then cut each in half, or even in quarters if they're very big.

- Throw them in a deep bowl and toss with olive oil, salt, pepper and any other spices you like. We sometimes toss them in red pepper and cumin!

- Pour them out onto a greased baking sheet making sure to leave a little bit a room between them. They don't all need to be on the same side, they'll all roast up nicely even if they look messy on that sheet.

- Place the baking sheet into the oven and bake for about 30 minutes. Halfway through, reach in to the oven and give the baking sheet a good shake so that the brussels sprouts rotate a little.

- While the brussels sprouts are baking, fry up as much bacon as you'd like. We use 2 pieces for each person we're feeding.

- When the bacon is cooked to your liking, chop it up into small pieces, roughly a half inch big, You want them bite sized.

- When the brussels sprouts have shriveled a bit and blackened, they're ready! Take them out of the oven and toss them in the same deep bowl with the bacon bits.

BAKED BUTTER GARLIC SHRIMP

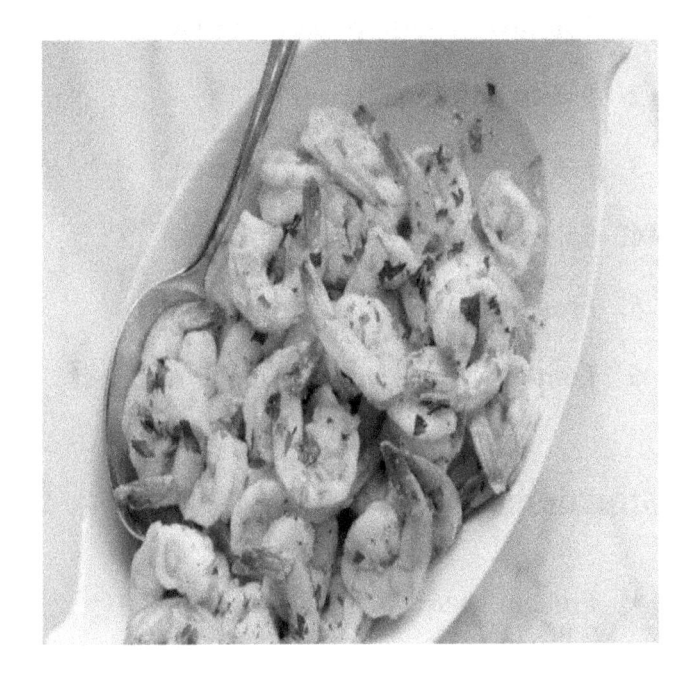

Quick and simple way to bake flavorful shrimp with no fuss. Garlic and butter shrimp. Toss with pasta or use butter sauce as a dip for crusty bread. Yum!

Prep time: 10 mins
Cook time: 20 mins
Carbs per meal:15g

Ingredients

1. 1 lb raw shrimp, peeled and cleaned
2. 5 tbsp softened butter
3. 3-4 large cloves garlic, crushed
4. Salt and fresh ground pepper
5. Fresh or dried parsley for garnish
6. Lemon wedges, for serving, if desired

Instructions

- Preheat oven to 425 degrees .
- Smear butter evenly over the bottom of the baking dish and then sprinkle the crushed garlic over the butter.
- Add the shrimp, trying not to overlap if possible.
- Sprinkle everything with salt and pepper.

- Bake for 7 minutes and then stir/turn the shrimp and bake for 7-10 more minutes, or until shrimp is done.

- Garnish with parsley, if desired, and squeeze a lemon wedge over it, if desired.

- Serve as a side with steak, or toss the cooked shrimp and butter sauce with pasta. If you do this, cook the pasta while the shrimp is cooking for a quick meal.

- Serve onto plates and give one last sprinkle of salt! Enjoy

ONE-PAN EGG & VEG BRUNCH

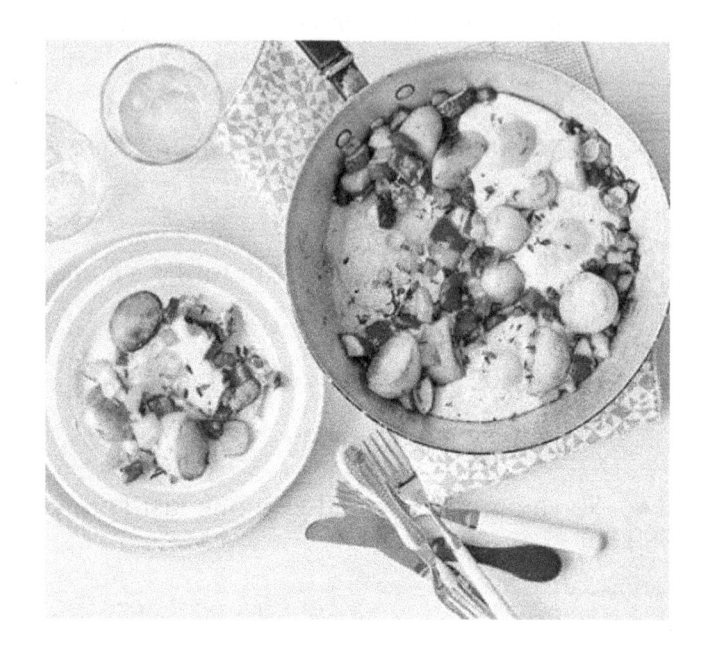

PREP: 5 MINS
COOK: 25 MINS
CARBS PER MEAL: 15g

INGREDIENTS:

1. 300g baby new potatoes, halved
2. ½ tbsp rapeseed oil
3. 1 knob of butter

4. 1 courgette, cut into small chunks
5. 1 yellow pepper, cut into small chunks
6. red pepper, cut into small chunks
7. spring onions, finely sliced
8. 1 garlic clove, crushed
9. 1 sprig thyme, leaves picked
10. 4 eggstoast, to serve

INSTRUCTIONS:

- Boil the new potatoes for 8 mins, then drain.
- Heat the oil and butter in a large non-stick frying pan, then add the courgette, peppers, potatoes and a little salt and pepper. Cook for 10 mins, stirring from time to time until everything is starting to brown. Add the spring onions, garlic and thyme and cook for 2 mins more.

- Make four spaces in the pan and crack in the eggs. Cover with foil or a lid and cook for around 4 mins, or until the eggs are cooked (with the yolks soft for dipping into). Sprinkle with more thyme leaves and ground black pepper if you like. Serve with toast.

PASTA WITH SALMON & PEAS

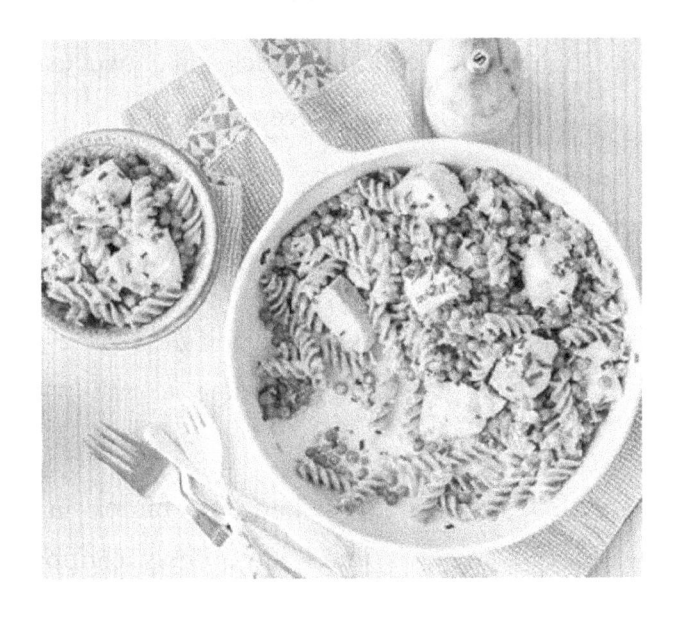

PREP: 15 MINS
COOK: 12 MINS - 15MINS
CARBS PER MEAL: 44g

INGREDIENTS:

1. 240g wholewheat fusilli knob of butter
2. large shallot, finely chopped
3. 140g frozen peas

4. skinless salmon fillets, cut into chunks

5. 140g low fat crème fraîche

6. ½ low salt vegetable stock cube (we used Kallo) small bunch chives, snipped

INSTRUCTIONS:

- Bring a pan of water to the boil and cook 240g whole wheat fusilli according to the pack instructions.

- Meanwhile, heat a knob of butter in a saucepan, then add 1 large finely chopped shallot and cook for 5 mins or until softened.

- Add 140g frozen peas, 2 skinless salmon fillets, cut into chunks, 140g low fat crème fraîche and 50ml water. Crumble in ½ low salt vegetable stock cube.

- Cook for 3-4 mins until cooked through, stir in small bunch snipped chives and some black pepper. Then stir through to coat the pasta. Serve in bowls.

PAPPARDELLE BROAD BEAN CARBONARA

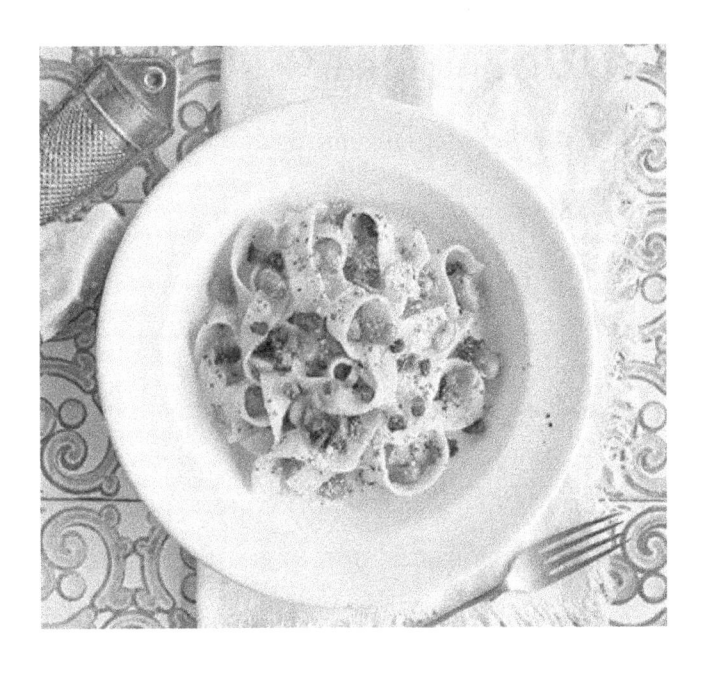

PREP: 10 MINS
COOK: 20 MINS
CARBS PER MEAL: 39g

INGREDIENTS:

1. 85g pancetta

2. 100g podded and skinned broad bean(about 400g unpodded)
3. 2 egg yolks
4. 2 tbsp double cream
5. 1 tbsp wholegrain mustard
6. 200g pappardelle pasta
7. 50g parmesan, grated

INSTRUCTIONS:

- Bring a large pan of salted water to the boil. While the water boils, heat a frying pan and sizzle the pancetta for 8 mins until crisp, then throw the broad beans into the pan with the pancetta fat. In a small bowl, beat the egg yolks with the cream and mustard, then season with lots of black pepper.

- Cook the pasta following pack instructions. Drain the pasta, saving some of the water, and toss through the pancetta in the frying pan. Tip in the egg and cream mix, and stir to coat, adding a splash of the reserved water, if needed. Toss half of the grated Parmesan through, so the sauce clings to the pasta, then scatter with the remaining Parmesan.

TOMATOES STUFFED WITH PESTO RICE

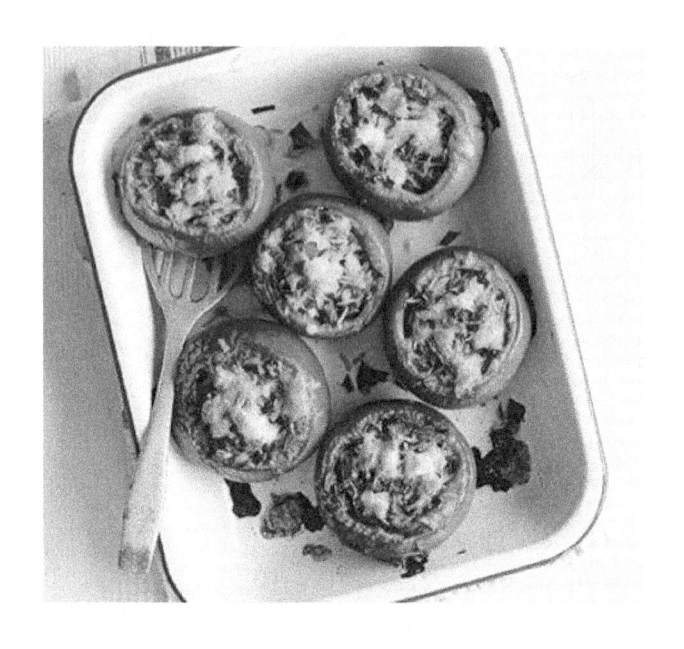

PREP: 10 MINS
COOK: 20 MINS
CARBS PER MEAL: 36g

INGREDIENTS:

1. 6 large beef tomatoes
2. 250g pack microwave rice

3. 3 tbsp vegetarian pesto (use Sacla organic basil pesto)
4. 100g grated mozzarella
5. 80g bag spinach, roughly chopped
6. 1 tbsp olive oil

INSTRUCTIONS:

- Heat oven to 200C/180C fan/gas 6. Slice the tops off the tomatoes and set aside. Scoop out the insides with a teaspoon, keeping the tomatoes intact. Discard the tomato flesh, but roughly chop the tomato tops. Heat the rice following pack instructions and tip into a bowl. Mix in the chopped tomato, the pesto, three-quarters of the mozzarella, the spinach and seasoning.

- Spoon the rice mixture into the tomatoes and pack tightly into a casserole dish. Sprinkle with the remaining cheese, drizzle with a little olive oil and bake for 20 mins until soft and bubbling.

HERB-AND-MUSTARD SIRLOIN WITH BAKED POTATOES

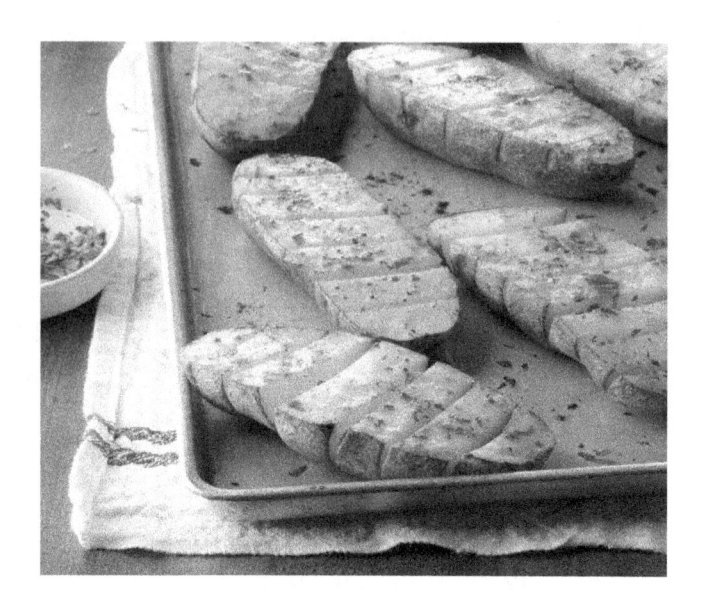

PREP: 10 MIN
COOK: 20 MIN
CARB PER MEAL: 31g

INGREDIENTS

1. 4 small russet potatoes, scrubbed

2. 1/2 pounds sirloin steak (1/2 inch thick)

3. tablespoons spicy mustard, plus more for serving
4. 2 teaspoons crumbled herbes de Provence
5. 5 tablespoons unsalted butter
6. Kosher salt and freshly ground pepper
7. 2 tablespoons chopped fresh chives or scallion greens

INSTRUCTIONS:

- Pierce the potatoes a few times with a fork, then microwave until soft, about 15 minutes.

- Meanwhile, pierce both sides of the steak with a fork. Mix the mustard and herbes de Provence in a bowl and rub all over the steak.

- Heat a large cast-iron skillet over medium-high heat. Add 1 tablespoon butter; as soon as it melts, add the steak and sear on one side until browned, about 7 minutes. Turn and brown the other side, about 4 more minutes for medium-rare. Transfer the steak to a cutting board, season with salt and pepper, and top with 1 tablespoon butter. Let rest at least 5 minutes.

- Return the skillet to medium-high heat. Add the potatoes and turn to coat on all sides with the pan juices. Cook until the skins are slightly crisp, about 3 minutes.

- Mix the remaining 3 tablespoons butter with the chives and season with salt. Thinly slice the steak on the bias. Serve with the potatoes, chive butter and mustard.

CHICKEN-AND-CHEESE ENCHILADAS

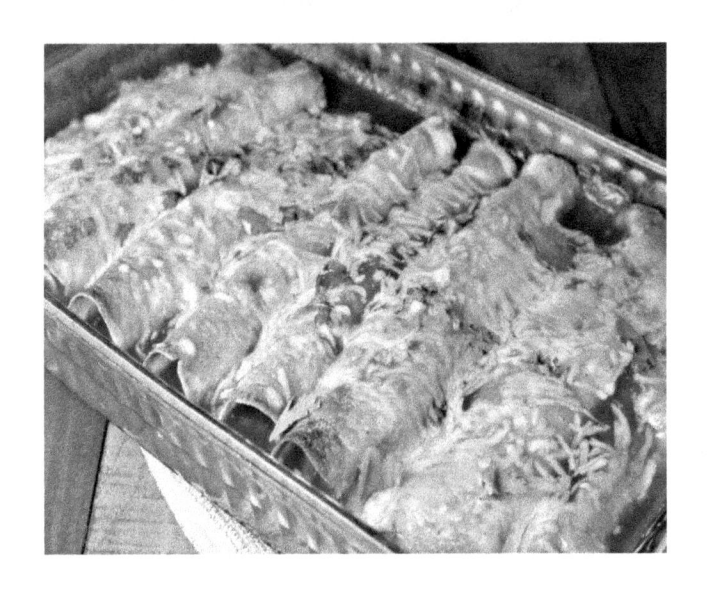

PREP: 15 MIN
COOK: 15 MIN
CARB PER MEAL: 46g

INGREDIENTS

1. 1 small red onion, halved

2. 1 1/2 pounds tomatillos, husked and rinsed

3. 1 to 2 serrano chile peppers, stemmed and seeded

4. 1/2 cup low-sodium chicken broth

5. Kosher salt

6. Pinch of sugar

7. 8 corn tortillas

8. 3 cups shredded rotisserie chicken

9. 2 1/2 cups shredded mozzarella and/or Monterey Jack cheese

10. 1/3 cup fresh cilantro

11. 2 tablespoons extra-virgin olive oil, plus more for greasing

12. 3/4 cup crumbled queso fresco or feta cheese

INSTRUCTIONS:

- Preheat the broiler. Slice half of the onion into thin rings and set aside. Place the other onion half, tomatillos and serranos on a foil-lined baking sheet and broil until the vegetables are soft and slightly brown, 7 to 10 minutes, turning as needed. Transfer the vegetables and any liquid to a blender, add the broth and puree. Season with 1/2 teaspoon salt and the sugar.

- Meanwhile, stack the tortillas, wrap in a damp paper towel and microwave just until warm and soft, 1 minute; keep covered. Toss the chicken with 2 cups shredded cheese in a bowl. Spoon a portion of the chicken mixture down the middle of each tortilla. Add a few cilantro leaves and roll up. Place the enchiladas side by side in a lightly oiled 9-by-13-inch baking dish and brush with the 2 tablespoons olive oil. Broil until crisp and golden, 3 minutes.

- Pour the tomatillo sauce over the enchiladas and top with the remaining 1/2 cup shredded cheese. Return to the oven and broil until the cheese is bubbly and golden brown, 3 to 5 minutes. Garnish with the onion rings, queso fresco and any remaining cilantro.

PITA PIZZAS

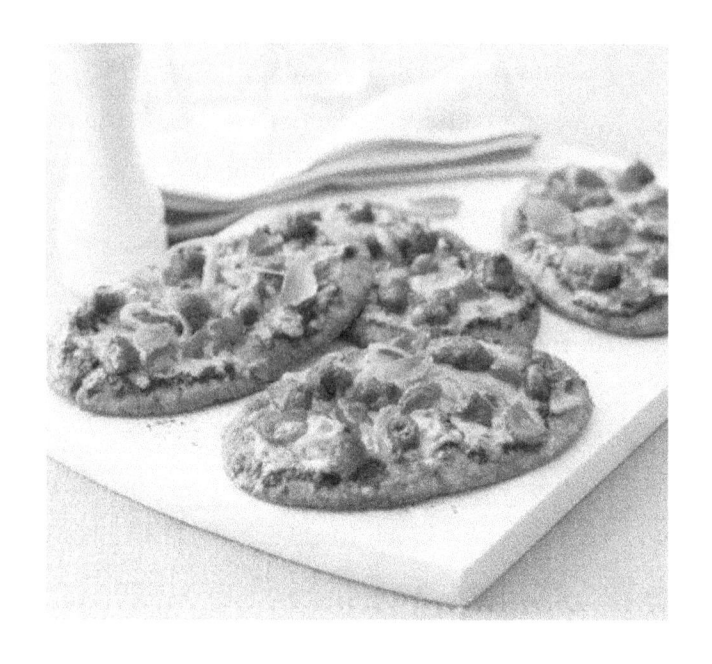

PREP: 5 MIN
COOK: 25 MIN
CARB PER MEAL: 46g

INGREDIENTS

1. 3 medium tomatoes

2. 1 tablespoon extra-virgin olive oil, plus more for brushing and drizzling

3. Kosher salt and freshly ground pepper

4. 3 cups baby arugula

5. 1/2 cup pitted kalamata olives, roughly chopped

6. 1 tablespoon fresh rosemary, roughly chopped

7. 1 large red onion, cut into 1-inch-thick rounds

8. 4 6-to-8-inch pocketless pitas

9. 1/2 cup ricotta cheese

10. 1/4 pound part-skim mozzarella cheese, diced

11. Pinch of red pepper flakes

INSTRUCTIONS:

- Core the tomatoes and halve them crosswise, then squeeze the juices and seeds into a large bowl. Whisk in 1 tablespoon olive oil and season with salt and pepper. Add the arugula but don't toss; set aside. Dice the tomatoes and toss in a separate bowl with the olives and rosemary.

- Preheat a grill to medium high. Brush the onion rounds with olive oil and season with salt. Grill until soft, 3 to 4 minutes per side. Transfer to a plate and separate the rings. Reduce the grill heat to medium.

- Brush both sides of the pitas with olive oil and grill until marked, 2 to 3 minutes per side. Top with some of the tomato-olive mixture, ricotta, mozzarella and onion. Cover and grill until the cheese melts, 2 to 3 minutes.

- Toss the arugula with the dressing and pile on top of the pitas. Season with salt and the red pepper flakes and drizzle with olive oil.

ROASTED BRUSSELS SPROUTS WITH BACON

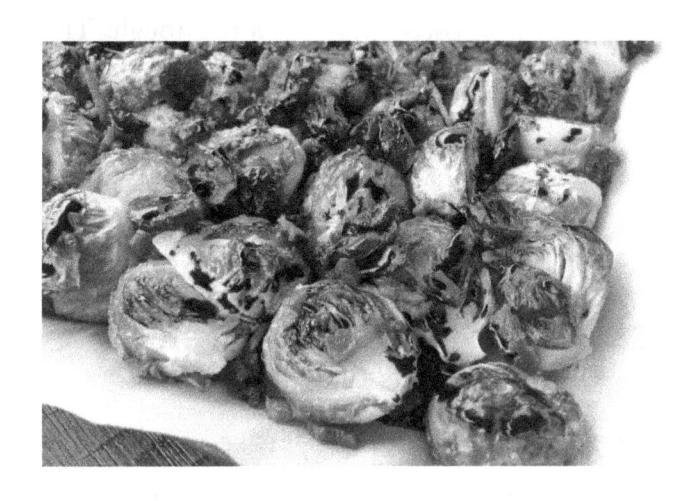

PREP TIME:5MINUTES
COOK TIME:25MINUTES
CARBS PER MEAL: 4g

INGREDIENTS

1. lb brussels sprouts
2. tbsp olive oil 8 strips bacon salt

pepper

INSTRUCTIONS:

- Preheat the oven to 375°F and cut the ends off of each brussels sprout, it's too tough. Then cut each in half, or even in quarters if they're very big.

- Throw them in a deep bowl and toss with olive oil, salt, pepper and any other spices you like. We sometimes toss them in red pepper and cumin!

- Pour them out onto a greased baking sheet making sure to leave a little bit a room between them. They don't all need to be on the same side, they'll all roast up nicely even if they look messy on that sheet.

- Place the baking sheet into the oven and bake for about 30 minutes. Halfway through, reach in to the oven and give the baking sheet a good shake so that the brussels sprouts rotate a little.

- While the brussels sprouts are baking, fry up as much bacon as you'd like. We use 2 pieces for each person we're feeding.

- When the bacon is cooked to your liking, chop it up into small pieces, roughly a half inch big, You want them bite sized.

- When the brussels sprouts have shriveled a bit and blackened, they're ready! Take them out of the oven and toss them in the same deep bowl with the bacon bits.

Serve onto plates and give one last sprinkle of salt! Enjoy!

Cauliflower Toast with Avocado

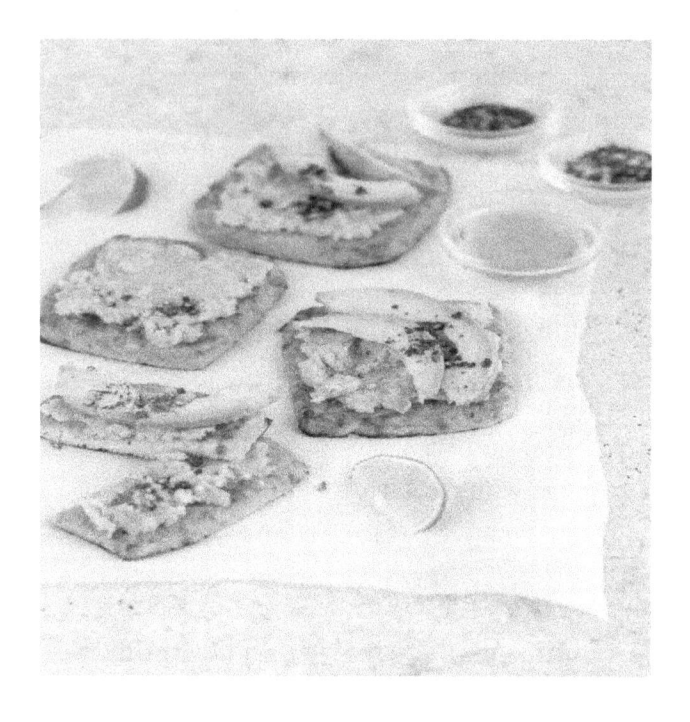

PREP: 10mins cook: 20mins carbs per MEAL:6.5g

INGREDIENTS:

1. 1 small head cauliflower (grated)

2. 1 large egg

3. **1/2 cup mozzarella cheese**

4. **1/2 teaspoon garlic powder**

5. **1 medium avocado (pitted and chopped)**

6. **1 tablespoon fresh lime juice**

7. **salt and pepper**

INSTRUCTIONS:

- Preheat the oven to 425°F and line a baking sheet with parchment or foil.
- Place the cauliflower in a microwave-safe bowl and heat on high for 8 minutes.
- After the cauliflower has cooled completely, spread on paper towels to drain and press with a clean towel to remove excess moisture.

- Put the cauliflower back in the bowl and stir in the egg, mozzarella cheese, and garlic powder.

- Season with salt and pepper and stir until well combined.

- Spoon the mixture onto the baking sheet in four rounded squares, as evenly as possible.

- Bake for 18 to 20 minutes until golden brown on the edges.

- Mash the avocado with the lime juice and a pinch of salt and pepper.

- Spread the avocado onto the cauliflower toast to serve. Makes 2 servings.

- For leftovers, prepare the cauliflower toast as directed and prepare the avocado mash fresh.

One-pot paprika cod and chickpeas

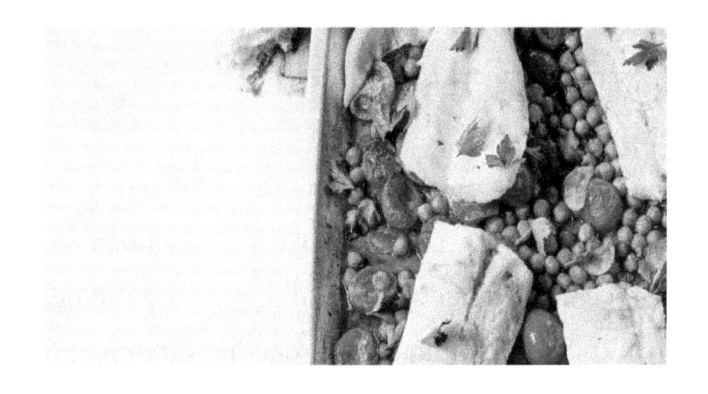

Prep time: 10 Minutes
Cook time: 20 minutes
Carbs per meal: 11.7

Ingredients:

1. garlic 1 clove, finely sliced   red chilli 1, finely sliced (optional)   baby plum tomatoes 300g, halved   chickpeas 400g tin, drained and rinsed   olive oil 3 tbsp   smoked paprika 1 tsp

2. cod loin fillets 4 pieces (about 125g each)   flat-leaf parsley a small bunch, chopped

lemon wedges to serve   crusty bread to serve

INSTRUCTIONS:

- Heat the oven to 190C/fan 170C/gas 5. Put the garlic, chilli (if using), tomatoes and chickpeas in a baking dish and add the olive oil and paprika. Toss together then roast for 10 minutes. Sit the cod on top, season, then put back in the oven for another 10-15 minutes or until the cod is cooked through and flakes easily. Scatter with parsley and serve with lemon wedges and crusty bread.

Zucchini & Sausage Stovetop Casserole

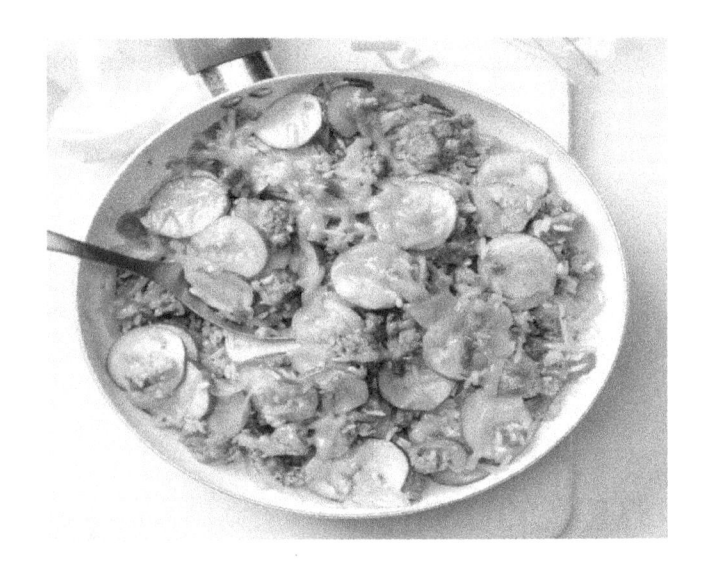

Prep: 10minutes
Cook:20min
Carbs per meal: 24g

Ingredients

1. 1 pound bulk pork sausage
2. 1 tablespoon canola oil
3. 3 medium zucchini, thinly sliced

4. 1 medium onion, chopped
5. 1 can (14-1/2 ounces) stewed tomatoes, cut up
6. 1 package (8.8 ounces) ready-to-serve long grain rice
7. 1 teaspoon prepared mustard
8. 1/2 teaspoon garlic salt
9. 1/4 teaspoon pepper
10. 1 cup shredded sharp cheddar cheese

INSTRUCTIONS

- In a large skillet, cook sausage over medium heat 5-7 minutes or until no longer pink, breaking into crumbles. Drain and remove sausage from pan.
- In same pan, heat oil over medium heat. Add zucchini and onion; cook and stir 5-7 minutes or until tender. Stir in sausage, tomatoes, rice, mustard, garlic salt and pepper. Bring to a

boil. Reduce heat; simmer, covered, 5 minutes to allow flavors to blend.

- Remove from heat; sprinkle with cheese. Let stand, covered, 5 minutes or until cheese is melted.
- Nutrition Facts
- 1-1/3 cups: 394 calories, 26g fat (9g saturated fat), 60mg cholesterol, 803mg sodium, 24g carbohydrate (6g sugars, 2g fiber), 16g protein.

Steak & Mushroom Stroganoff

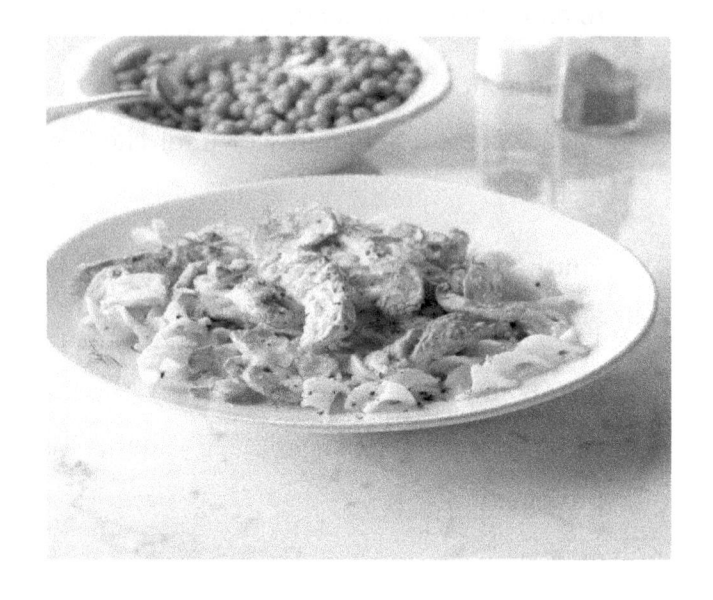

Prep/Total Time: 30 minutes
Carbs per meal: 34g

INGREDIENTS:

1. 6 cups uncooked egg noodles (about 12 ounces)

2. 1 beef top sirloin steak (1-1/2 pounds), cut into 2x1/2-in. strips

3. 1 tablespoon canola oil
4. 1/2 teaspoon salt
5. 1/2 teaspoon pepper
6. 2 tablespoons butter
7. **1 pound sliced fresh mushrooms**
8. 2 shallots, finely chopped
9. 1/2 cup beef broth
10. **1 tablespoon snipped fresh dill**
11. **1 cup sour cream**

INSTRUCTIONS:

- Cook noodles according to package directions; drain.

- Meanwhile, toss beef with oil, salt and pepper. Place a large skillet over medium-high heat; saute half of the beef until browned, 2-3 minutes. Remove from pan; repeat with remaining beef.

- In same pan, heat butter over medium-high heat; saute mushrooms until lightly browned, 4-6 minutes. Add shallots; cook and stir until tender, 1-2 minutes. Stir in broth, dill and beef; heat through. Reduce heat to medium; stir in sour cream until blended. Serve with noodles.

Parmesan Chicken with Lemon Rice

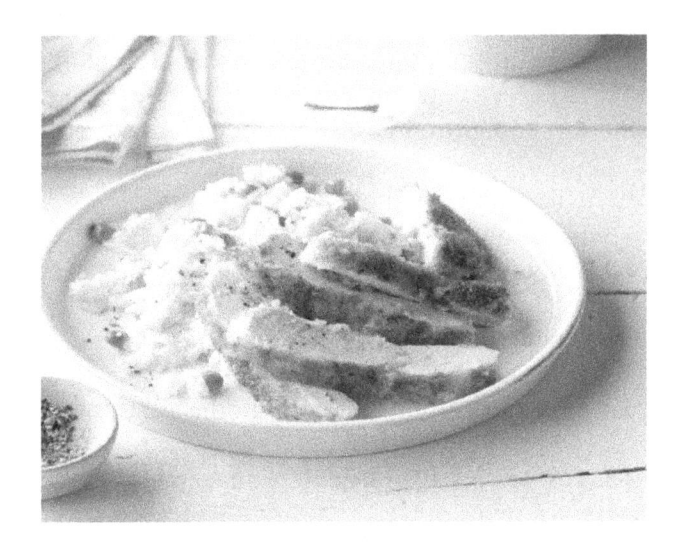

Prep/Total time: 30minutes
Carbs per meal:55g

Ingredients

1. 2 cups reduced-sodium chicken broth
2. 2 tablespoons lemon juice
3. 1 cup uncooked long grain rice
4. 1/2 cup chopped onion

5. 1 large Eggland's Best egg

6. 2 tablespoons fat-free milk

7. 3/4 cup panko (Japanese) bread crumbs

8. 2/3 cup grated Parmesan cheese, divided

9. 1 teaspoon dried oregano

10. 1 pound boneless skinless chicken breasts

11. 2 tablespoons olive oil

12. 1 cup frozen peas (about 4 ounces), thawed

13. 1/4 teaspoon grated lemon zest • Freshly ground pepper, optional

INSTRUCTIONS:

- In a saucepan, bring broth and lemon juice to a boil. Stir in rice and onion; return to a boil. Reduce heat; simmer, covered, until liquid is almost absorbed and rice is tender, 15-20 minutes.

- Meanwhile, in a shallow bowl, whisk together egg and milk. In another bowl, toss bread crumbs with 1/3 cup cheese and oregano. Pound chicken breasts with a meat mallet to 1/4-in. thickness. Dip in egg mixture, then in crumb mixture to coat both sides.

- In a large skillet, heat oil over medium heat. Cook chicken until golden brown and chicken is no longer pink, 2-3 minutes per side.

- When rice is cooked, gently stir in peas; cook, covered, until heated through, 1-2 minutes. Stir in lemon zest and remaining cheese. Cut chicken into slices; serve with rice. If desired, sprinkle with pepper.

Grilled Salmon with Chorizo-Olive Sauce

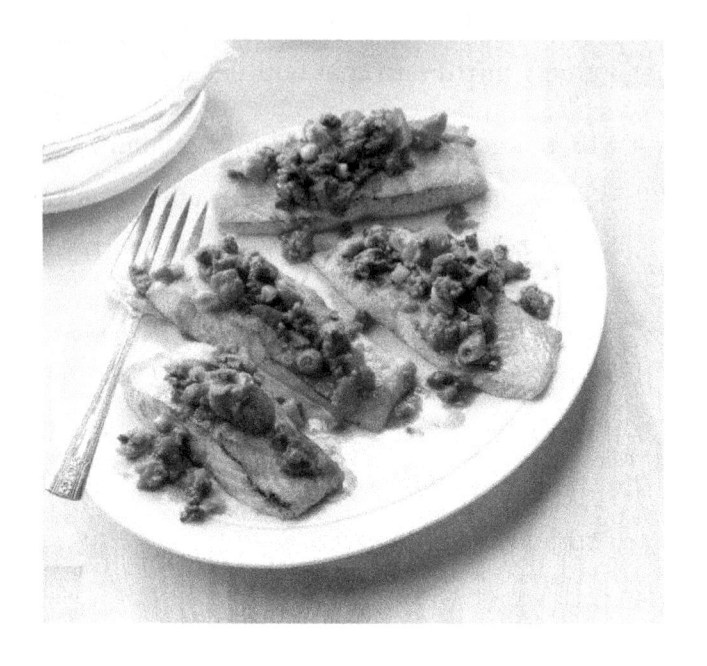

Prep/Total Time: 25 min.
Carbs per meal: 7g

Ingredients

1. 3 links (3 to 4 ounces each) fresh chorizo
2. 4 green onions, chopped

3. 2 garlic cloves, minced
4. 1 can (14-1/2 ounces) diced tomatoes, drained
5. 1/4 cup chopped pitted green olives
6. 1/2 teaspoon grated orange zest
7. 1/4 teaspoon salt
8. 1/4 teaspoon pepper
9. 4 salmon fillets (6 ounces each)

INSTRUCTIONS:

- Remove chorizo from casings. In a large ovenproof skillet on a stove or grill, cook and stir chorizo, green onions and garlic over medium-high heat, crumbling sausage. Cook until sausage is no longer pink, 4-6 minutes; drain.

- Reduce heat to medium. Add tomatoes, olives and orange zest; stir to combine. Sprinkle salt and pepper over salmon.

- On a greased grill rack, grill salmon, covered, over medium heat 3-4 minutes per side, or until fish just begins to flake easily with a fork. Top with chorizo mixture.

Beef & Bacon Gnocchi Skillet

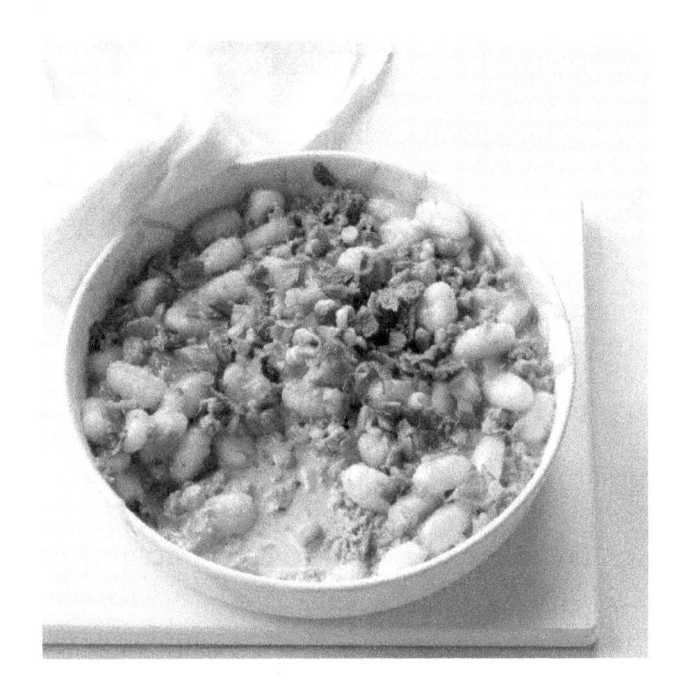

Prep/Total Time: 30 min
Carbs per meal:35g

Ingredients

1. 1 package (16 ounces) potato gnocchi
2. 1-1/4 pounds lean ground beef (90% lean)
3. 1 medium onion, chopped

4. 8 cooked bacon strips, crumbled and divided

5. 1 cup water

6. 1/2 cup heavy whipping cream

7. 1 tablespoon ketchup

8. 1/4 teaspoon salt

9. 1/4 teaspoon pepper

10. 1-1/2 cups shredded cheddar cheese

11. 1/2 cup chopped tomatoes

12. 2 green onions, sliced

13. Preheat broiler. Cook gnocchi according to package directions; drain.

Instruction

- Meanwhile, in a large cast-iron or other ovenproof skillet, cook beef and onion, crumbling beef, over medium heat until no longer pink, 4-6 minutes. Drain.

- Stir in half of the bacon; add gnocchi, water, cream and ketchup. Bring to a boil. Cook, stirring, over medium heat until sauce has thickened, 3-4 minutes. Add salt and pepper. Sprinkle with cheese.

- Broil 3-4 Min. from heat until cheese has melted, 1-2 minutes. Top with tomatoes, green onions and remaining bacon.

Chili Dog Pizza

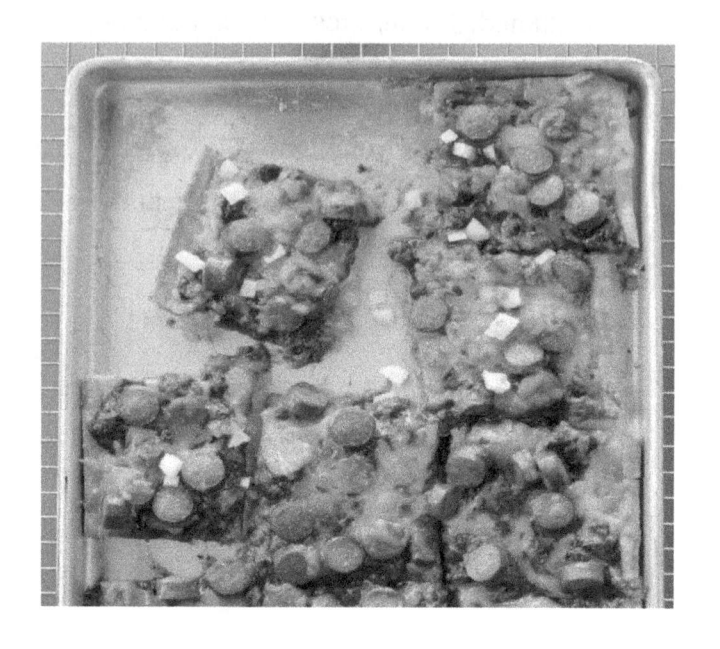

Prep/Total Time: 25 min.
Carbs per meal: 28g

Ingredients

1. 1 tube (11 ounces) refrigerated thin pizza crust
2. 1/2 cup yellow mustard
3. 1 can (15 ounces) chili with beans

4. 6 hot dogs, sliced
5. 2 cups shredded cheddar cheese
6. Chopped onion and sweet pickle relish, optional

INSTRUCTIONS

- Preheat oven to 425°. Unroll and press dough into bottom of a greased 15x10x1-in. baking pan. Bake until edges are lightly browned, 5-7 minutes.

- Spread with mustard; top with chili, hot dogs and cheese. Bake until crust is golden and cheese is melted, 10-15 minutes. If desired, sprinkle with onion and relish.

Chicken Tamale Bake

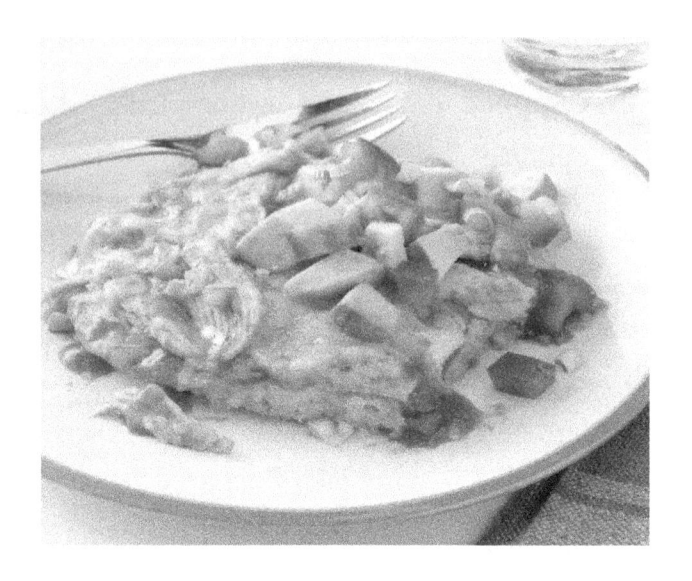

Prep: 10 min. Bake: 25 min. + standing
Carbs per meal: 35g

Ingredients

1. 1 large egg, lightly beaten
2. 1 can (14-3/4 ounces) cream-style corn
3. 1 package (8-1/2 ounces) cornbread/muffin mix

4. 1 can (4 ounces) chopped green chilies

5. 1/3 cup 2% milk

6. 1/4 cup shredded Mexican cheese blend

7. TOPPING:

8. 2 cups coarsely shredded cooked chicken

9. 1 can (10 ounces) enchilada sauce

10. 1 teaspoon ground cumin

11. 1/2 teaspoon onion powder

12. 1-3/4 cups shredded Mexican cheese blend

13. Chopped green onions, tomatoes and avocado, optional

INSTRUCTIONS:

- Preheat oven to 400°. In a large bowl, combine the first six ingredients; stir just until dry ingredients are moistened. Transfer to a greased 13x9-in. baking dish. Bake until light golden brown and a toothpick inserted in center comes out clean, 15-18 minutes.

- In a large skillet, combine chicken, enchilada sauce, cumin and onion powder; bring to a boil, stirring occasionally. Reduce heat; simmer, uncovered, 5 minutes. Spread over cornbread layer; sprinkle with cheese.

- Bake until cheese is melted, 10-12 minutes longer. Let stand 10 minutes before serving. If desired, top with green onions, tomatoes and avocado.

Ginger Halibut with Brussels Sprouts

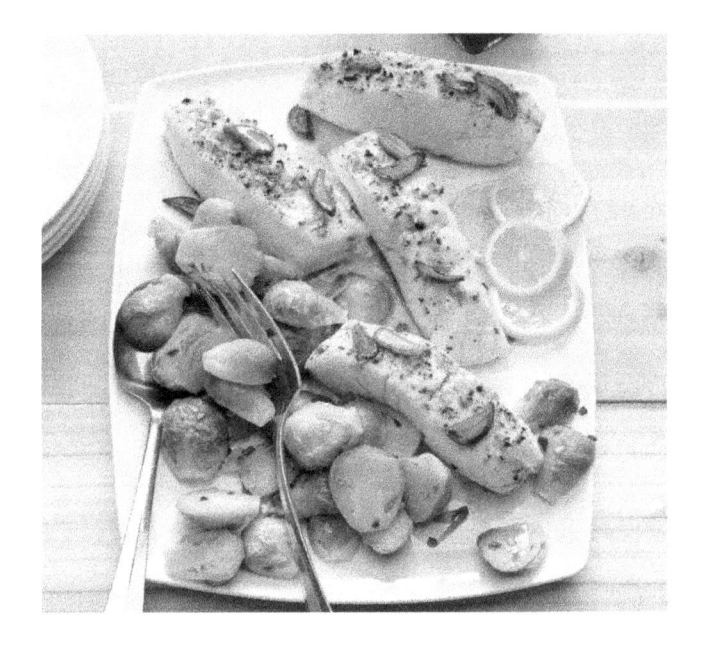

Prep/Total Time: 25 min.
Carbs per meal: 7g

Ingredients

1. 4 teaspoons lemon juice

2. 4 halibut fillets (4 to 6 ounces each)

3. 1 teaspoon minced fresh gingerroot

4. 1/4 to 3/4 teaspoon salt, divided

5. 1/4 teaspoon pepper

6. 1/2 cup water

7. 10 ounces (about 2-1/2 cups) fresh Brussels sprouts, halved

8. Crushed red pepper flakes

9. 1 tablespoon canola oil

10. 5 garlic cloves, sliced lengthwise

11. 2 tablespoons sesame oil

12. 2 tablespoons soy sauce

13. Lemon slices, optional

INSTRUCTIONS:

- Brush lemon juice over halibut fillets. Sprinkle with minced ginger, 1/4 teaspoon salt and pepper.

- Place fish on an oiled grill rack, skin side down. Grill, covered, over medium heat (or broil 6 in. from heat) until fish just begins to flake easily with a fork, 6-8 minutes.

- In a large skillet, bring water to a boil over medium-high heat. Add Brussels sprouts, pepper flakes and, if desired, remaining salt. Cook, covered, until tender, 5-7 minutes. Meanwhile, in a small skillet, heat oil over medium heat. Add garlic; cook until golden brown. Drain on paper towels.

- Drizzle sesame oil and soy sauce over halibut. Serve with Brussels sprouts; sprinkle with fried garlic. If desired, serve with lemon slices.

One-Pot Spinach Beef Soup

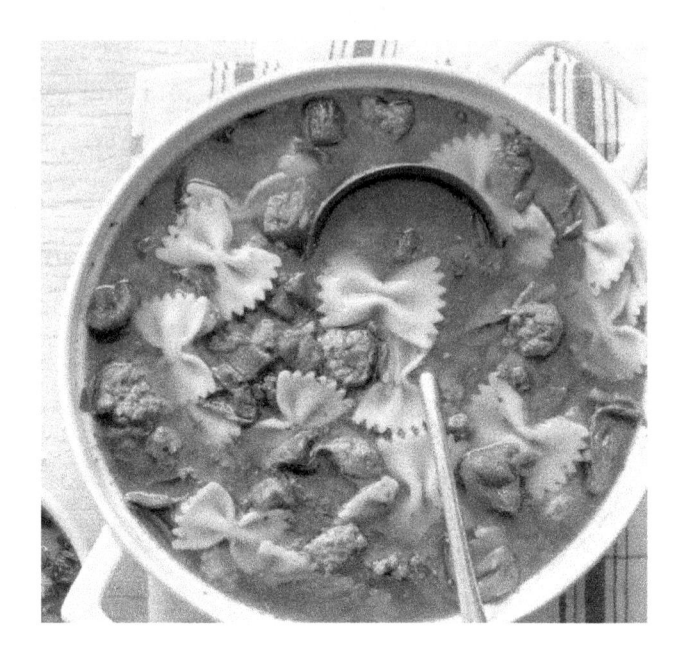

Prep/Total Time: 30 min.
Carbs per meal:30g

Ingredients

1. 1 pound ground beef
2. 3 garlic cloves, minced

3. 2 cartons (32 ounces each) reduced-sodium beef broth
4. 2 cans (14-1/2 ounces each) diced tomatoes with green pepper, celery and onion, undrained
5. 1 teaspoon dried basil
6. 1/2 teaspoon pepper
7. 1/2 teaspoon dried oregano
8. 1/4 teaspoon salt
9. 3 cups uncooked bow tie pasta
10. 4 cups fresh spinach, coarsely chopped
11. Grated Parmesan cheese

INSTRUCTIONS:

- In a 6-qt. stockpot, cook beef and garlic over medium heat until beef is no longer pink, breaking up beef into crumbles, 6-8 minutes; drain. Stir in broth, tomatoes and seasonings;

bring to a boil. Stir in pasta; return to a boil. Cook, uncovered, until pasta is tender, 7-9 minutes.

- Stir in spinach until wilted. Sprinkle servings with cheese.

Bucatini with Sausage & Kale

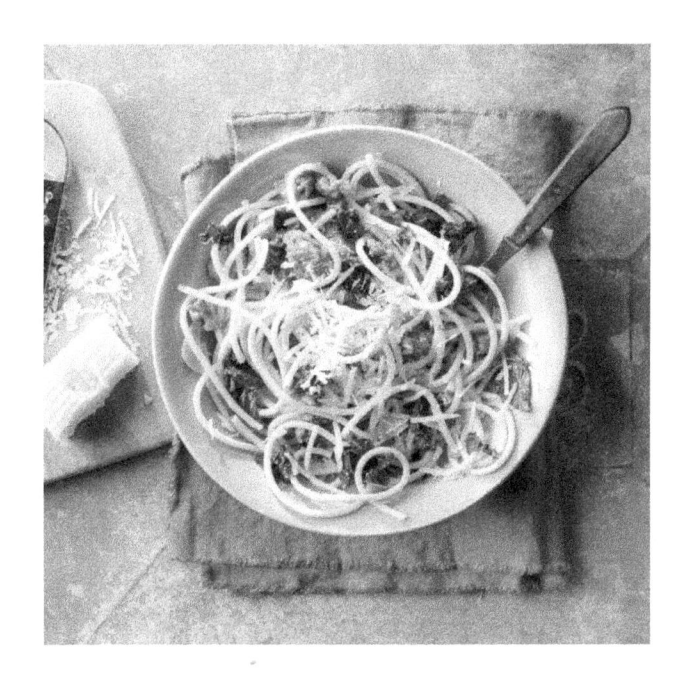

*Prep/Total Time: 30 min.
Carbs per meal: 43g*

INGREDIENTS:

1. package (12 ounces) bucatini pasta or fettuccine

2. teaspoons plus 3 tablespoons olive oil, divided

3. 1 pound regular or spicy bulk Italian sausage

4. 5 garlic cloves, thinly sliced

5. 8 cups chopped fresh kale (about 5 ounces)

6. 3/4 teaspoon salt

7. 1/4 teaspoon pepper

8. Shredded Romano cheese

INSTRUCTIONS:

- Cook pasta according to package directions, decreasing time by 3 minutes. Drain, reserving 2 cups pasta water. Toss pasta with 2 teaspoons oil.

- In a 6-qt. stockpot, cook sausage over medium heat until no longer pink, 5-7 minutes, breaking sausage into large crumbles. Add garlic and remaining oil; cook and stir 2 minutes. Stir in kale, salt and pepper; cook, covered, over medium-low heat until kale is tender, about 10 minutes, stirring occasionally.

- Add pasta and reserved pasta water; bring to a boil. Reduce heat; simmer, uncovered, until pasta is al dente and liquid is absorbed, about 3 minutes, tossing to combine. Sprinkle with cheese.

BBQ Hot Dog & Potato Packs

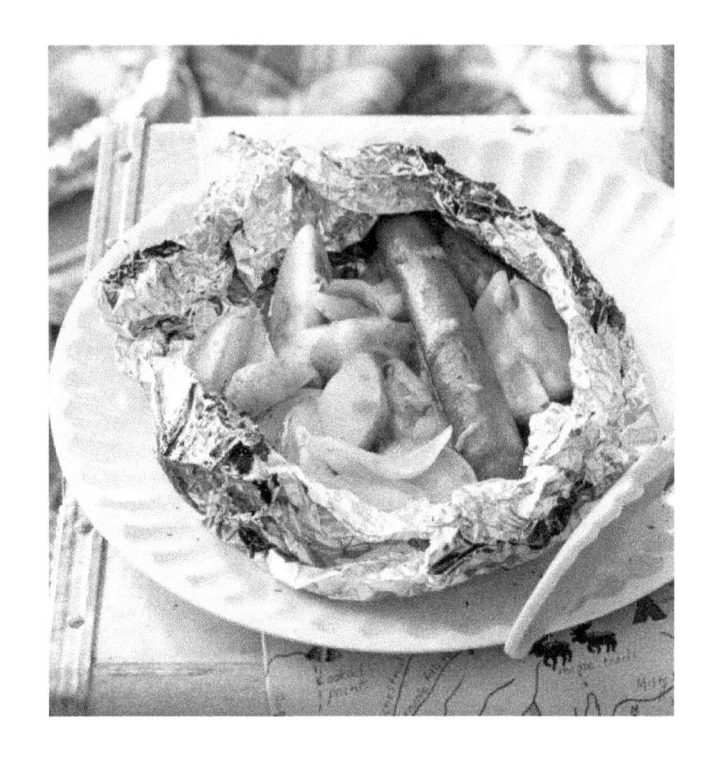

*Prep/Total Time: 20 min.
Carbs per meal:25g*

INGREDIENTS:

1. 1 package (20 ounces) refrigerated red potato wedges

2. **4 hot dogs**

3. **1 small onion, cut into wedges**

4. **1/4 cup shredded cheddar cheese**

5. **1/2 cup barbecue sauce**

INSTRUCTIONS:

- Divide potato wedges among four pieces of heavy-duty foil (about 18 in. square). Top each with a hot dog, onion wedges and cheese. Drizzle with barbecue sauce. Fold foil around mixture, sealing tightly.

- Grill, covered, over medium heat 10-15 minutes or until heated through. Open foil carefully to allow steam to escape.

Grilled Chicken Chopped Salad

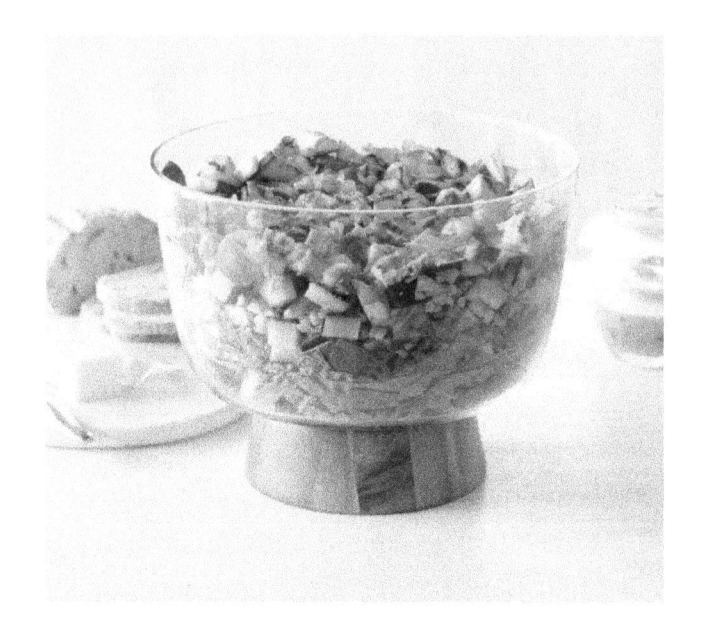

*Prep/Total Time: 30 min.
Carbs per meal:21g*

Ingredients

1. 1 pound chicken tenderloins
2. 6 tablespoons zesty Italian salad dressing, divided
3. 2 medium zucchini, quartered lengthwise

4. 1 medium red onion, quartered
5. 2 medium ears sweet corn, husks removed
6. 1 bunch romaine, chopped
7. 1 medium cucumber, chopped
8. Additional salad dressing, optional

INSTRUCTIONS:

- In a bowl, toss chicken with 4 tablespoons dressing. Brush zucchini and onion with remaining 2 tablespoons dressing.

- Place corn, zucchini and onion on a grill rack over medium heat; close lid. Grill zucchini and onion 2-3 minutes on each side or until tender. Grill corn 10-12 minutes or until tender, turning occasionally.

- Drain chicken, discarding marinade. Grill chicken, covered, over medium heat 3-4 minutes on each side or until no longer pink.

- Cut corn from cobs; cut zucchini, onion and chicken into bite-sized pieces. In a 3-qt. trifle bowl or other glass bowl, layer romaine, cucumber, grilled vegetables and chicken. If desired, serve with additional dressing.

Spicy Shrimp & Watermelon Kabobs

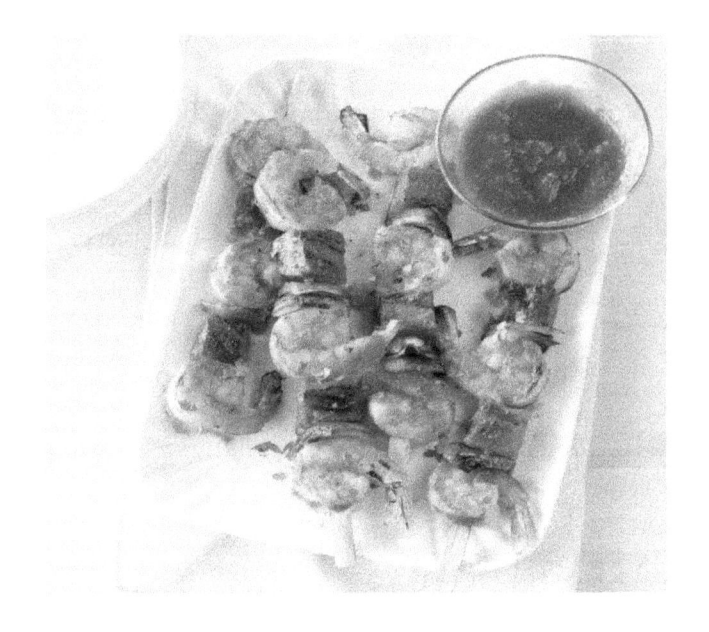

Prep/Total Time: 30 min.
Carbs per meal: 23g

Ingredients

1. 1 tablespoon reduced-sodium soy sauce
2. 1 tablespoon Sriracha chili sauce
3. 1 tablespoon honey

4. 1 garlic clove, minced

5. 4 cups cubed seedless watermelon (1 inch), divided

6. 1 pound uncooked shrimp (16-20 per pound), peeled and deveined

7. 1 medium red onion, cut into 1-inch pieces

8. 1/2 teaspoon sea salt

9. 1/4 teaspoon coarsely ground pepper

10. Minced fresh cilantro, optional

INSTRUCTIONS

- For glaze, place soy sauce, chili sauce, honey, garlic and 2 cups watermelon in a blender; cover and process until pureed. Transfer to a small saucepan; bring to a boil. Cook, uncovered, over medium-high heat until mixture is reduced by half, about 10 minutes. Reserve 1/4 cup glaze for serving.
- On four metal or soaked wooden skewers, alternately thread shrimp, onion and

remaining watermelon. Sprinkle with salt and pepper.

- Place kabobs on an oiled grill rack over medium heat. Grill, covered, 3-4 minutes on each side or until shrimp turns pink, brushing with remaining glaze during the last 2 minutes. If desired, sprinkle with cilantro. Serve with reserved glaze.

Health Tip: A serving of fruit with dinner? Check. Along with 20 percent of the daily value for vitamin C.

Pizza in a Bowl

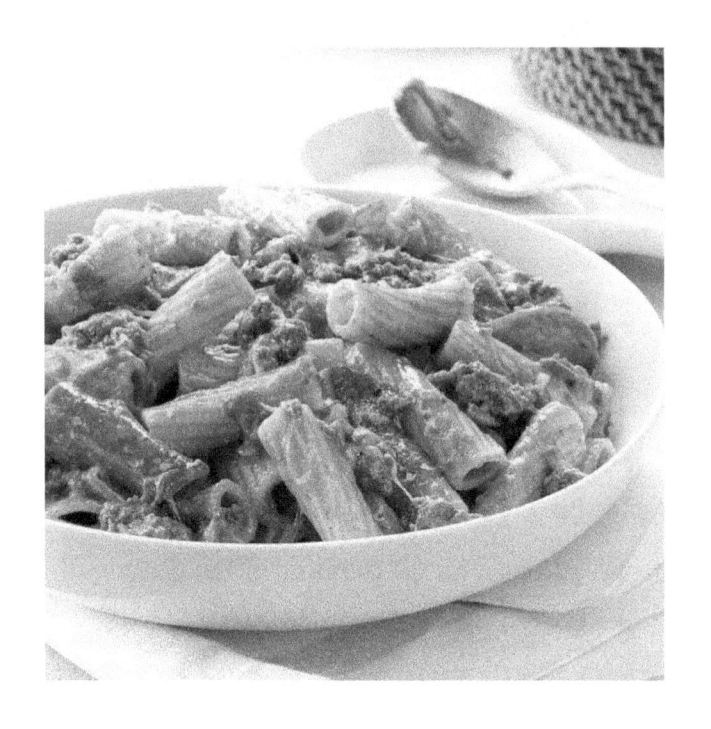

Prep/Total Time: 25 min.
Carbs per meal: 37g

Ingredients

1. 8 ounces uncooked rigatoni (about 3 cups)
2. 3/4 pound ground beef

3. 1/2 cup chopped onion
4. 1 can (15 ounces) pizza sauce
5. 2/3 cup condensed cream of mushroom soup, undiluted
6. 2 cups shredded part-skim mozzarella cheese
7. 1 package (3-1/2 ounces) sliced pepperoni
8. Chopped fresh basil or arugula, optional

INSTRUCTIONS:

- Cook rigatoni according to package directions; drain. Meanwhile, in a large skillet, cook beef and onion over medium heat 6-8 minutes or until beef is no longer pink, breaking up beef into crumbles; drain. Add pizza sauce, soup and cheese; cook and stir over low heat until cheese is melted.

- Add rigatoni and pepperoni to beef mixture. Heat through, stirring to combine. If desired, top with basil before serving.

Cauliflower & Tofu Curry

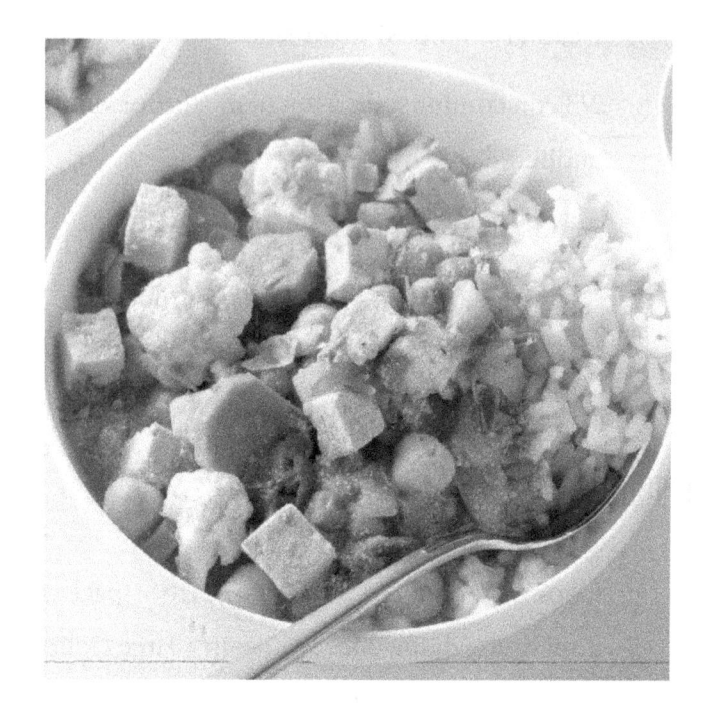

Prep/Total Time: 30 min.
Carbs per meal: 29g

Ingredients

1. 1 tablespoon olive oil
2. 2 medium carrots, sliced

3. 1 medium onion, chopped
4. 3 teaspoons curry powder
5. 1/4 teaspoon salt
6. 1/4 teaspoon pepper
7. 1 small head cauliflower, broken into florets (about 3 cups)
8. 1 can (14-1/2 ounces) fire-roasted crushed tomatoes
9. 1 package (14 ounces) extra-firm tofu, drained and cut into 1/2-inch cubes
10. 1 cup vegetable broth
11. 1 can (15 ounces) garbanzo beans or chickpeas, rinsed and drained
12. 1 can (13.66 ounces) coconut milk
13. 1 cup frozen peas
14. Hot cooked rice
15. Chopped fresh cilantro

INSTRUCTIONS:

- In a 6-qt. stockpot, heat oil over medium-high heat. Add carrots and onion; cook and stir until onion is tender, 4-5 minutes. Stir in seasonings.

- Add cauliflower, tomatoes, tofu and broth; bring to a boil. Reduce heat; simmer, covered, 10 minutes. Stir in garbanzo beans, coconut milk and peas; return to a boil. Reduce heat to medium; cook, uncovered, stirring occasionally, until slightly thickened and cauliflower is tender, 5-7 minutes.

- Serve with rice. Sprinkle with cilantro.

- Health Tip: Just one-half cup cooked cauliflower provides nearly half the daily value for vitamin C, not to mention sulfur-containing compounds that may help protect against certain cancers.

Lemon-Garlic Pork Chops

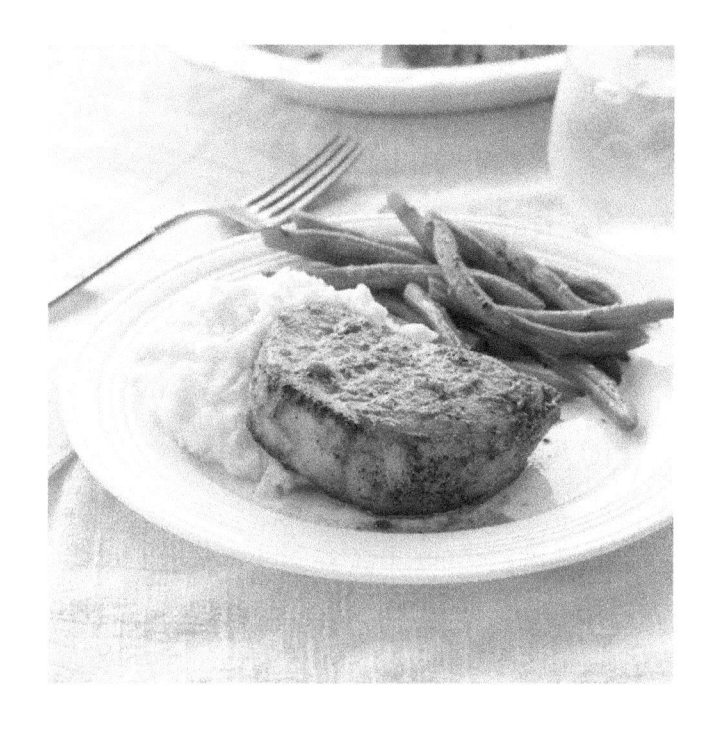

Prep/Total Time: 20 min
Carbs per meal: 2g

INGREDIENTS

1. **2 tablespoons lemon juice**

2. **2 garlic cloves, minced**

3. **1 teaspoon salt**

4. **1 teaspoon paprika**

5. **1/2 teaspoon pepper**

6. **1/4 teaspoon cayenne pepper**

7. **4 boneless pork loin chops (6 ounces each)**

INSTRUCTIONS:

- Preheat broiler. In a small bowl, mix the first six ingredients; brush over pork chops. Place in a 15x10x1-in. baking pan.

- Broil 4-5 in. from heat until a thermometer reads 145°, 4-5 minutes on each side. Let stand 5 minutes before serving.

Apple & Sweet Potato Quinoa

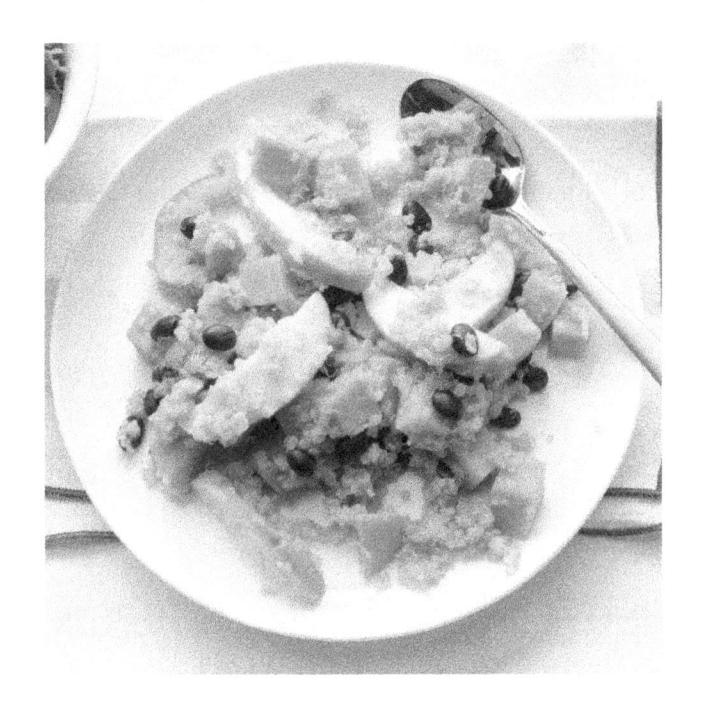

Prep/Total Time: 30 min.
Carbs per meal:76g

INGREDIENTS

1. 2-1/4 cups chicken or vegetable stock
2. 1 cup quinoa, rinsed

3. 2 tablespoons canola oil

4. 2 pounds sweet potatoes (about 3 medium), peeled and cut into 1/2-inch pieces

5. 2 shallots, finely chopped

6. 3 medium Gala or Honeycrisp apples, cut into 1/4-inch slices

7. 1/2 cup white wine or additional stock

8. 1/2 teaspoon salt

9. 1 can (15 ounces) black beans, rinsed and drained

INSTRUCTIONS:

- In a large saucepan, combine stock and quinoa; bring to a boil. Reduce heat; simmer, covered, 15-20 minutes or until liquid is almost absorbed. Remove from heat.

- Meanwhile, in a 6-qt. stockpot, heat oil over medium heat. Add sweet potatoes and shallots; cook and stir 5 minutes. Add apples;

cook and stir 68 minutes longer until potatoes and apples are tender.

- Stir in wine and salt. Bring to a boil; cook, uncovered, until wine is evaporated, about 1 minute. Stir in black beans and quinoa; heat through.

- Health Tip: Quinoa is one of the only plant foods that has all of the amino acids we need. Cook it up with gluten-free vegetable stock for a meatless meal that's also gluten-free.

Haddock with Lime-Cilantro Butter

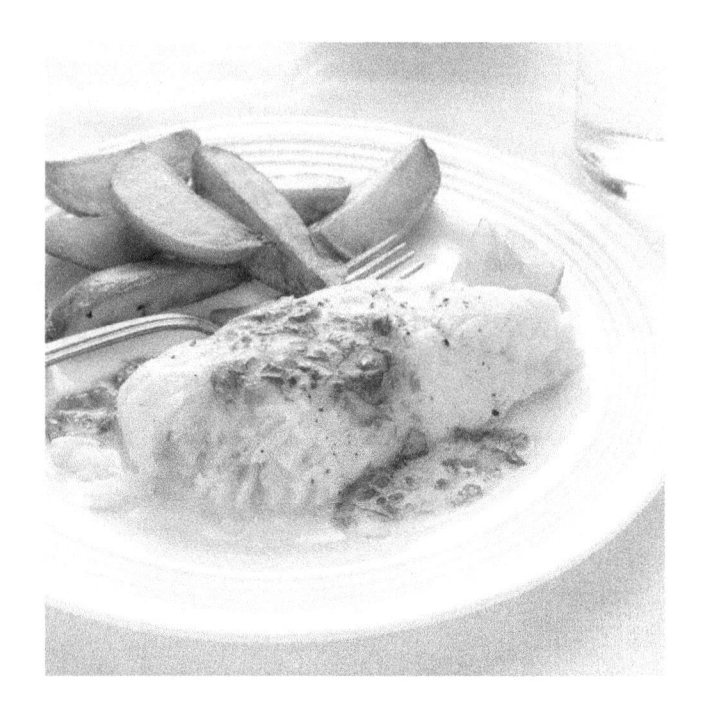

Prep/Total Time: 15 min.
Carbs per meal: 1g

INGREDIENTS

1. 4 haddock fillets (6 ounces each)
2. 1/2 teaspoon salt

3. 1/4 teaspoon pepper
4. 3 tablespoons butter, melted
5. 2 tablespoons minced fresh cilantro
6. 1 tablespoon lime juice • 1 teaspoon grated lime zest

INSTRUCTIONS:

- Preheat broiler. Sprinkle fillets with salt and pepper. Place on a greased broiler pan. Broil 4-5 in. from heat until fish flakes easily with a fork, 5-6 minutes.
- In a small bowl, mix remaining ingredients. Serve over fish.

Hoisin Turkey Lettuce Wraps

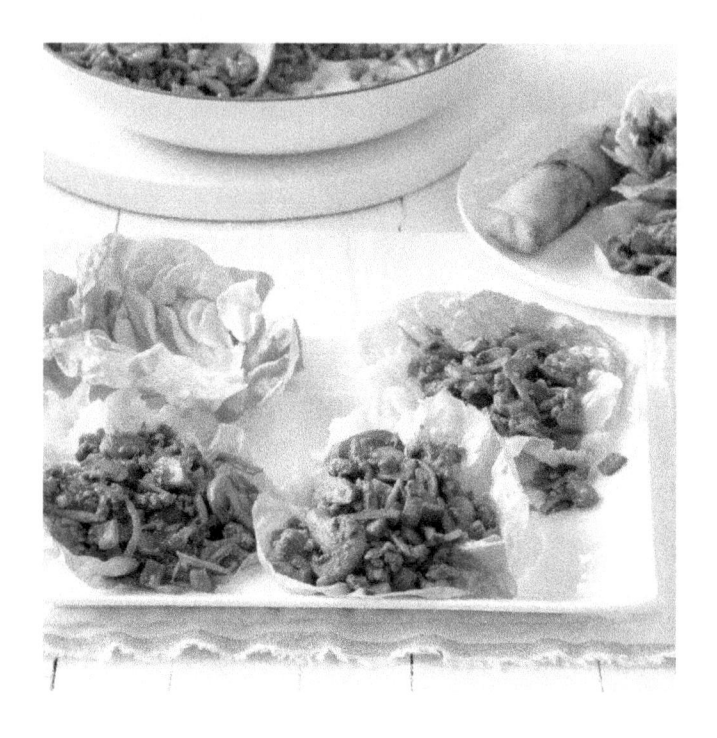

Prep/Total Time: 30 min.
Carbs per meal: 19g

INGREDIENTS

1. 1 pound lean ground turkey
2. 1/2 pound sliced fresh mushrooms

3. 1 medium sweet red pepper, diced
4. 1 medium onion, finely chopped
5. 1 medium carrot, shredded
6. 1 tablespoon sesame oil
7. 1/4 cup hoisin sauce
8. 2 tablespoons balsamic vinegar
9. 2 tablespoons reduced-sodium soy sauce
10. 1 tablespoon minced fresh gingerroot
11. 2 garlic cloves, minced • 8 Bibb or Boston lettuce leaves

INSTRUCTIONS:

- In a large skillet, cook and crumble turkey with vegetables in sesame oil over medium-high heat until turkey is no longer pink, 8-10 minutes, breaking up turkey into crumbles. Stir in hoisin sauce, vinegar, soy sauce, ginger and garlic; cook and stir over medium heat until sauce is slightly thickened, about 5 minutes. Serve in lettuce leaves.

Waffle-Iron Pizzas

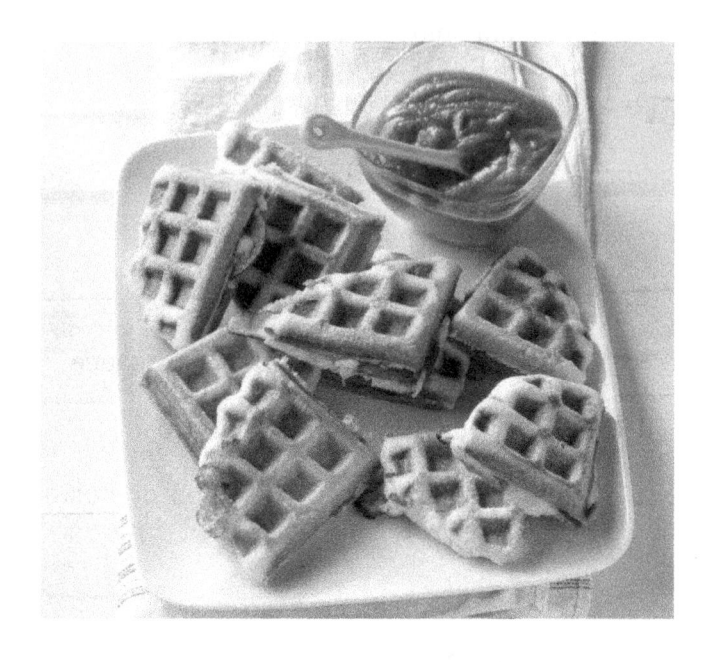

Prep/Total: 30 min.
Carbs per meal: 50g

INGREDIENTS

1. 1 package (16.3 ounces) large refrigerated buttermilk biscuits

2. 1 cup shredded part-skim mozzarella cheese

3. 24 slices turkey pepperoni (about 1-1/2 ounces)

4. 2 ready-to-serve fully cooked bacon strips, chopped

5. Pizza sauce, warmed

INSTRUCTIONS:

- Roll or press biscuits into 6-in. circles. On one biscuit, place 1/4 cup cheese, six slices pepperoni and a scant tablespoon chopped bacon to within 1/2 in. of edges. Top with a second biscuit, folding bottom edge over top edge and pressing to seal completely.

- Bake in a preheated waffle maker according to manufacturer's directions until golden brown, 4-5 minutes. Repeat with remaining ingredients. Serve with pizza sauce.

Southern Pork & Rice

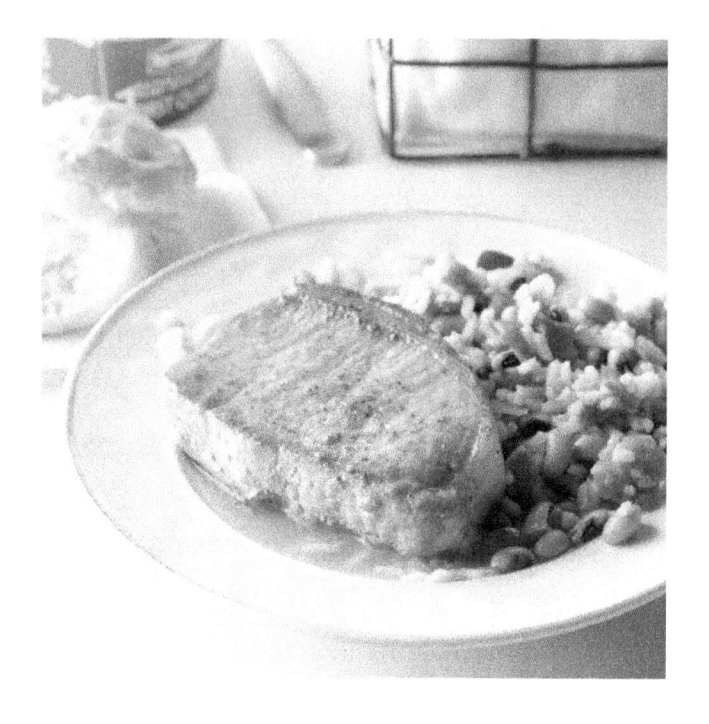

Prep/Total Time: 25 min.
Carbs per meal: 45g

INGREDIENTS

1. 4 boneless pork loin chops (6 ounces each)
2. 1 teaspoon seafood seasoning, divided

3. 1 tablespoon olive oil
4. 1 medium sweet red pepper, chopped
5. 1 medium onion, chopped
6. 2 teaspoons Worcestershire sauce
7. 1 can (15-1/2 ounces) black-eyed peas, rinsed and drained
8. 1 can (14-1/2 ounces) diced tomatoes with mild green chiles
9. 1 cup uncooked instant rice
10. 1 cup reduced-sodium chicken broth

INSTRUCTIONS

- Sprinkle pork with 3/4 teaspoon seafood seasoning. In a large skillet, heat oil over medium heat; brown chops on both sides. Remove from pan.
- Add pepper and onion to skillet; cook and stir until tender, 4-5 minutes. Stir in remaining

seafood seasoning, Worcestershire sauce, peas, tomatoes, rice and broth. Bring to a boil. Place chops over top. Reduce heat; simmer, covered, until a thermometer inserted in pork reads 145°, 2-3 minutes. Let stand, covered, 5 minutes before serving.

- Health tip: Make this meal gluten-free by using gluten-free broth and Worcestershire sauce.

Cheesy Chicken & Broccoli Orzo

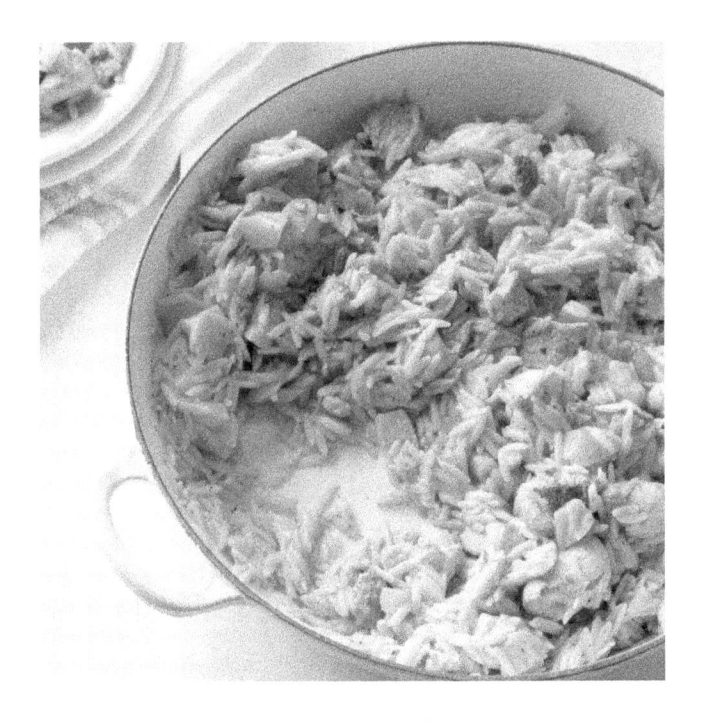

Prep/Total Time: 30 min
Carbs per meal: 38g

INGREDIENTS

1. 1-1/4 cups uncooked orzo pasta

2. 2 packages (10 ounces each) frozen broccoli with cheese sauce

3. 2 tablespoons butter

4. 1-1/2 pounds boneless skinless chicken breasts, cut into 1/2-inch cubes

5. 1 medium onion, chopped

6. 3/4 teaspoon salt

7. 1/2 teaspoon pepper

INSTRUCTIONS:

- Cook orzo according to package directions. Meanwhile, heat broccoli with cheese sauce according to package directions.

- In a large skillet, heat butter over medium heat. Add chicken, onion, salt and pepper; cook and stir 6-8 minutes or until chicken is no longer pink and onion is tender. Drain orzo. Stir orzo and broccoli with cheese sauce into skillet; heat through.

Apple, White Cheddar & Arugula Tarts

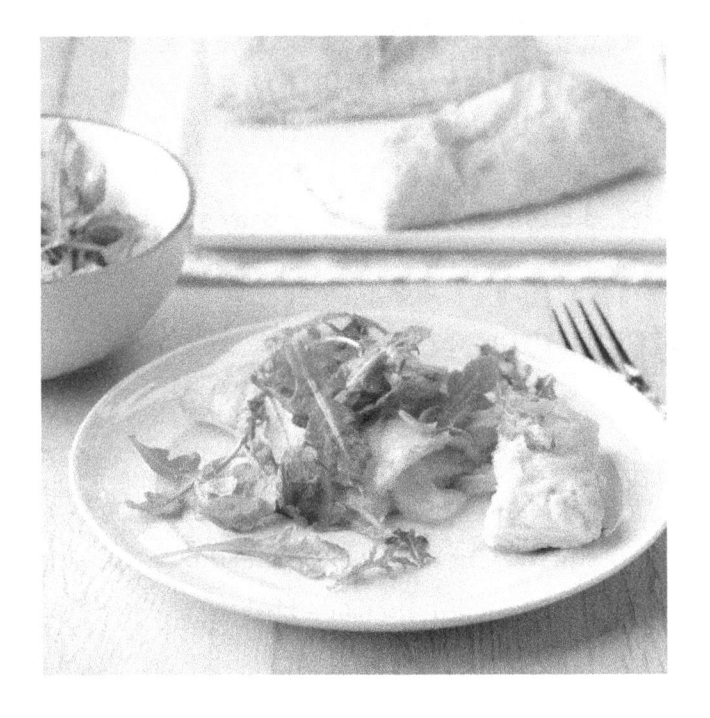

Prep/Total Time: 30 min
Carbs per meal: 46g

Ingredients

1. 1 sheet frozen puff pastry, thawed

2. 1 cup shredded white cheddar cheese

3. 2 medium apples, thinly sliced

4. 2 tablespoons olive oil

5. 1 tablespoon lemon juice

6. 3 cups fresh arugula or baby spinach

INSTRUCTIONS:

- Preheat oven to 400°. On a lightly floured surface, unfold puff pastry; roll into a 12-in. square. Cut pastry into four squares; place on a parchment paper-lined baking sheet.

- Sprinkle half of each square with cheese to within 1/4 in. of edges; top with apples. Fold pastry over filling. Press edges with a fork to seal. Bake 16-18 minutes or until golden brown.

- In a bowl, whisk oil and lemon juice until blended; add arugula and toss to coat. Serve with tarts.

Grilled Citrus Salmon

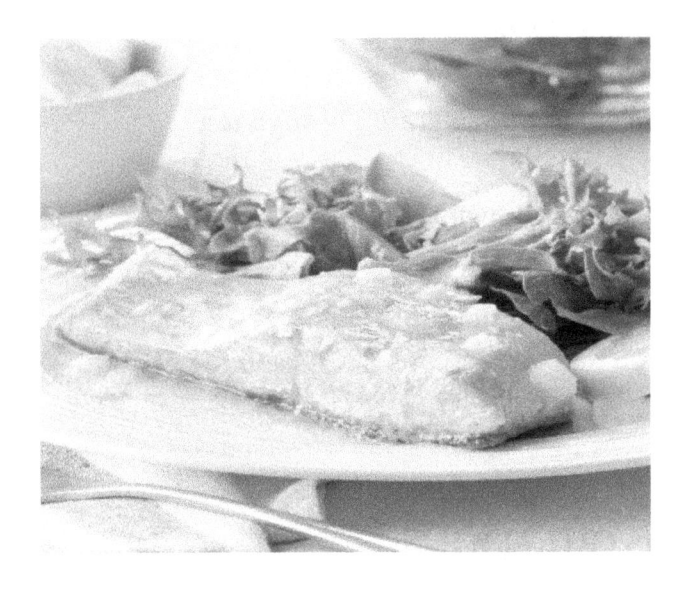

Prep/Total Time: 30 min.
Carbs per meal: 3g

Ingredients

1. **1/2 cup canola oil**

2. **1 medium onion, diced**

3. **2 tablespoons lemon juice**

4. 2 tablespoons orange juice

5. 1 teaspoon grated lemon zest

6. 1 teaspoon grated orange zest

7. 1 garlic clove, minced

8. 2 salmon fillets (about 1-1/2 pounds each)

9. orange or lemon slices, optional

INSTRUCTIONS:

- Combine the first seven ingredients in a jar with a tight-fitting lid; shake well. Grill salmon over medium heat, skin side down, for 15-20 minutes or until fish flakes easily with a fork. Baste every 5 minutes with citrus mixture. Garnish with orange or lemon slices if desired.

Zesty Grilled Chops

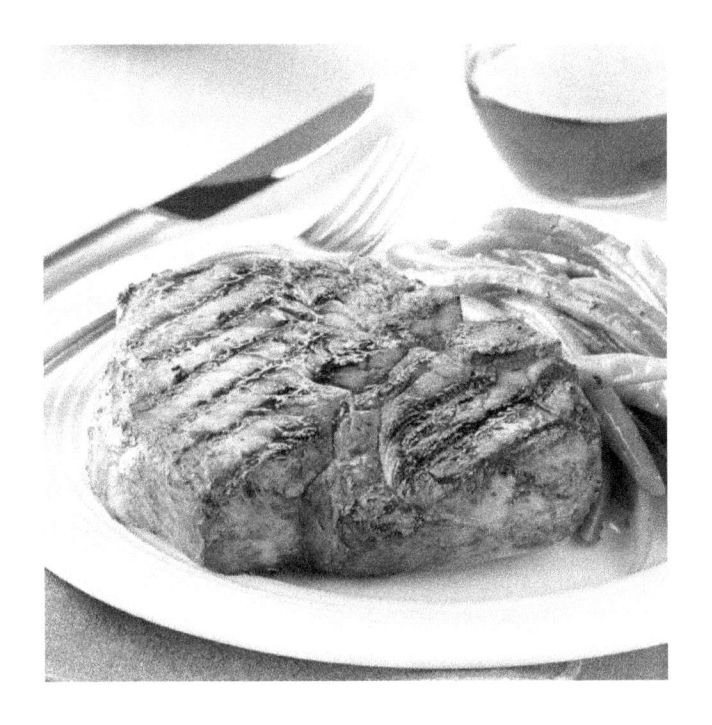

*Prep: 10 min. + marinating Grill: 10 min.
Carbs per meal: 1g*

Ingredients

1. 3/4 cup soy sauce
2. 1/4 cup lemon juice

3. 1 tablespoon chili sauce

4. 1 tablespoon brown sugar

5. 1 garlic clove, minced

6. 6 bone-in pork loin or rib chops (about 1-1/2 inches thick)

INSTRUCTIONS:

- In a large resealable plastic bag, combine first five ingredients; reserve 1/3 cup mixture for brushing over chops. Add pork chops to bag; seal bag and turn to coat. Refrigerate overnight.

- Drain pork, discarding marinade. Grill chops, covered, over medium heat or broil 4 in. from heat until a thermometer reads 145°, 6-8 minutes per side. Brush occasionally with reserved soy mixture during the last 5 minutes. Let stand 5 minutes before serving.

Caribbean Shrimp & Rice Bowl

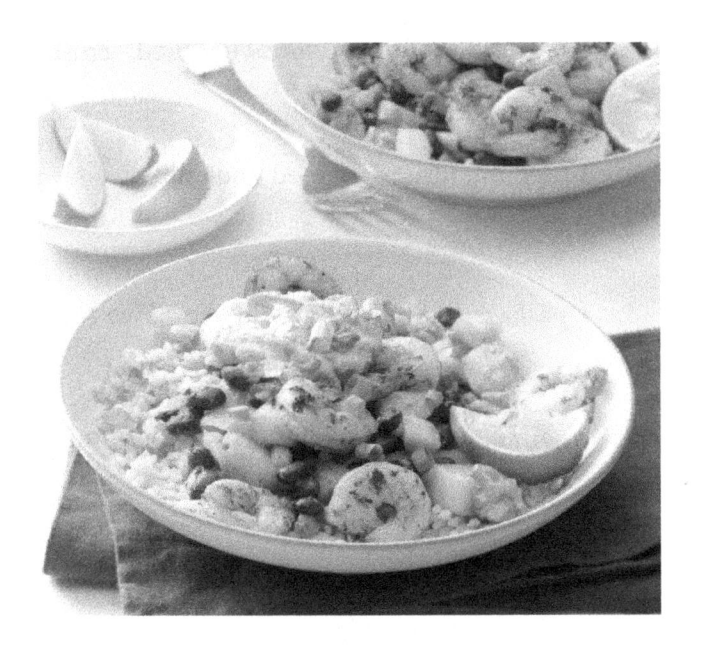

Prep/Total Time: 20 min.
Carbs per meal: 62g

Ingredients

1. 1 medium ripe avocado, peeled and pitted
2. 1/3 cup reduced-fat sour cream
3. 1/4 teaspoon salt

4. 1 can (15 ounces) black beans, rinsed and drained

5. 1 can (8 ounces) unsweetened crushed pineapple, undrained

6. 1 medium mango, peeled and cubed

7. 1/2 cup salsa

8. 1 package (8.8 ounces) ready-to-serve brown rice

9. 1 pound uncooked shrimp (31-40 per pound), peeled and deveined

10. 1 teaspoon Caribbean jerk seasoning

11. 1 tablespoon canola oil

12. 2 green onions, sliced

13. Lime wedges, optional

INSTRUCTIONS

- For avocado cream, mash avocado with sour cream and salt until smooth. In a small saucepan, combine beans, pineapple, mango and salsa; heat through, stirring occasionally. Prepare rice according to package directions.

- Toss shrimp with jerk seasoning. In a large skillet, heat oil over mediumhigh heat. Add shrimp; cook and stir until shrimp turn pink, 2-3 minutes.

- Divide rice and bean mixture among four bowls. Top with shrimp and green onions. Serve with avocado cream and, if desired, lime wedges.

Sausage-Stuffed Butternut Squash

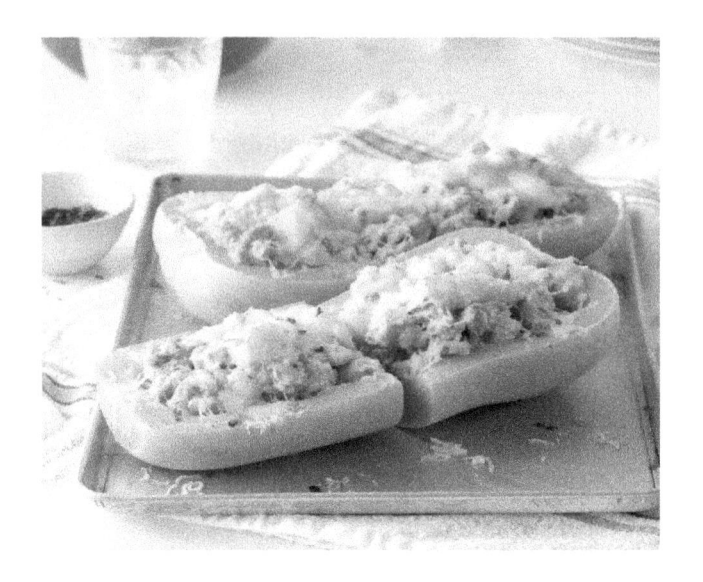

Prep/Total Time: 30 min
Carbs per meal: 44g

Ingredients

1. 1 medium butternut squash (about 3 pounds)
2. 1 pound Italian turkey sausage links, casings removed
3. 1 medium onion, finely chopped

4. 4 garlic cloves, minced

5. 1/2 cup shredded Italian cheese blend

6. Crushed red pepper flakes, optional

INSTRUCTIONS

- Preheat broiler. Cut squash lengthwise in half; discard seeds. Place squash in a large microwave-safe dish, cut side down; add 1/2 in. of water. Microwave, covered, on high until soft, 20-25 minutes. Cool slightly.

- Meanwhile, in a large nonstick skillet, cook and crumble sausage with onion over medium-high heat until no longer pink, 5-7 minutes. Add garlic; cook and stir 1 minute.

- Leaving 1/2-in.-thick shells, scoop pulp from squash and stir into sausage mixture. Place squash shells on a baking sheet; fill with sausage mixture. Sprinkle with cheese.

- Broil 4-5 in. from heat until cheese is melted, 1-2 minutes. If desired, sprinkle with pepper flakes. To serve, cut each half into two portions.

Health Tip: Butternut squash is an excellent source of vitamin A in the form of beta-carotene. It's important for normal vision and a healthy immune system, and it helps the heart, lungs and kidneys function properly.

Spicy Chicken Nuggets

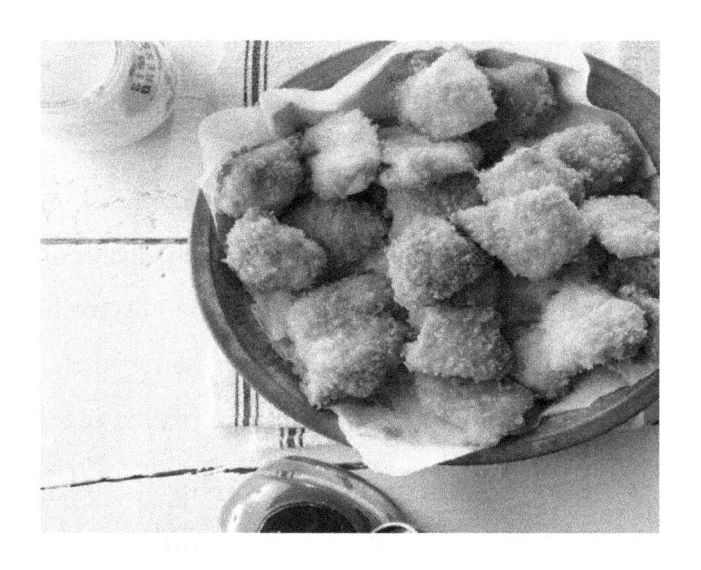

Prep/Total Time: 30 min.
Carbs per meal: 13g

Ingredients

1. 1-1/2 cups panko (Japanese) bread crumbs

2. 1-1/2 cups grated Parmesan cheese

3. 1/2 teaspoon ground chipotle pepper, optional

4. 1/4 cup butter, melted

5. 1-1/2 pounds boneless skinless chicken thighs, cut into 1-1/2-inch pieces

INSTRUCTIONS

- Preheat oven to 400°. In a shallow bowl, mix bread crumbs, cheese and, if desired, chipotle pepper. Place butter in a separate shallow bowl. Dip chicken pieces in butter, then in crumb mixture, patting to help coating adhere.

- Place chicken on a greased 15x10x1-in. baking pan; sprinkle with remaining crumb mixture. Bake 20-25 minutes or until no longer pink.

Scallops with Wilted Spinach

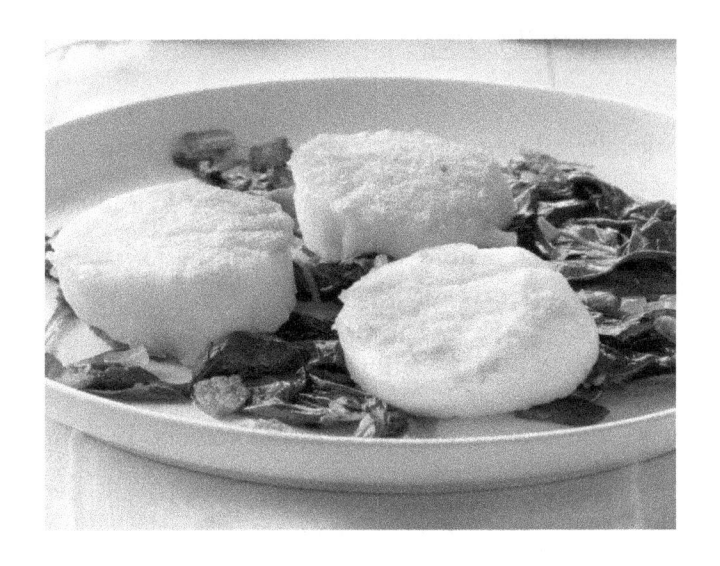

*Prep/Total Time: 25 min.
Carbs per meal: 12g*

Ingredients

1. 4 bacon strips, chopped
2. 12 sea scallops (about 1-1/2 pounds), side muscles removed
3. 2 shallots, finely chopped
4. 1/2 cup white wine or chicken broth

5. 8 cups fresh baby spinach (about 8 ounces)

INSTRUCTIONS:

- In a large nonstick skillet, cook bacon over medium heat until crisp, stirring occasionally. Remove with a slotted spoon; drain on paper towels. Discard drippings, reserving 2 tablespoons. Wipe skillet clean if necessary.

- Pat scallops dry with paper towels. In same skillet, heat 1 tablespoon drippings over medium-high heat. Add scallops; cook until golden brown and firm, 2-3 minutes on each side. Remove from pan; keep warm.

- Heat remaining drippings in same pan over medium-high heat. Add shallots; cook and stir until tender, 2-3 minutes. Add wine; bring to a boil, stirring to loosen browned bits from pan. Add spinach; cook and stir until wilted, 1-2 minutes. Stir in bacon. Serve with scallops.

Mom's Spanish Rice

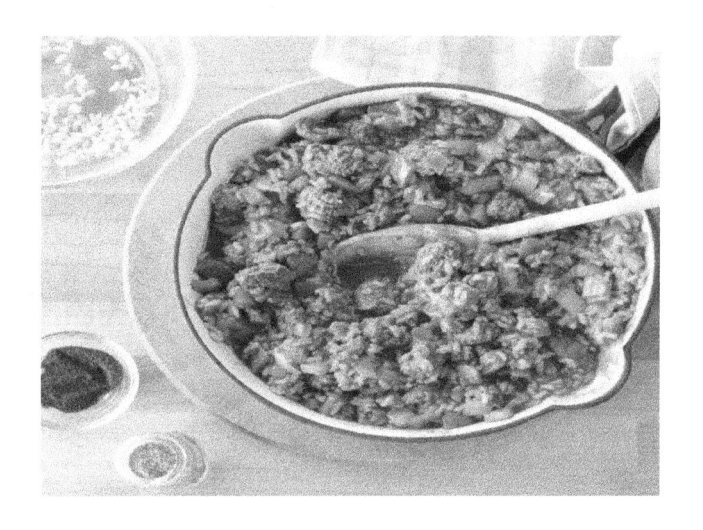

Prep/Total Time: 20 min
Carbs per meal: 49g

Ingredients

1. 1 pound lean ground beef (90% lean)
2. 1 large onion, chopped
3. 1 medium green pepper, chopped
4. 1 can (15 ounces) tomato sauce

5. 1 can (14-1/2 ounces) no-salt-added diced tomatoes, drained
6. 1 teaspoon ground cumin
7. 1 teaspoon chili powder
8. 1/2 teaspoon garlic powder
9. 1/4 teaspoon salt
10. 2-2/3 cups cooked brown rice

INSTRUCTIONS:

- In a large skillet, cook beef, onion and pepper over medium heat 6-8 minutes or until beef is no longer pink and onion is tender, breaking up beef into crumbles; drain.

- Stir in tomato sauce, tomatoes and seasonings; bring to a boil. Add rice; heat through, stirring occasionally.

Easy Buffalo Chicken Dip

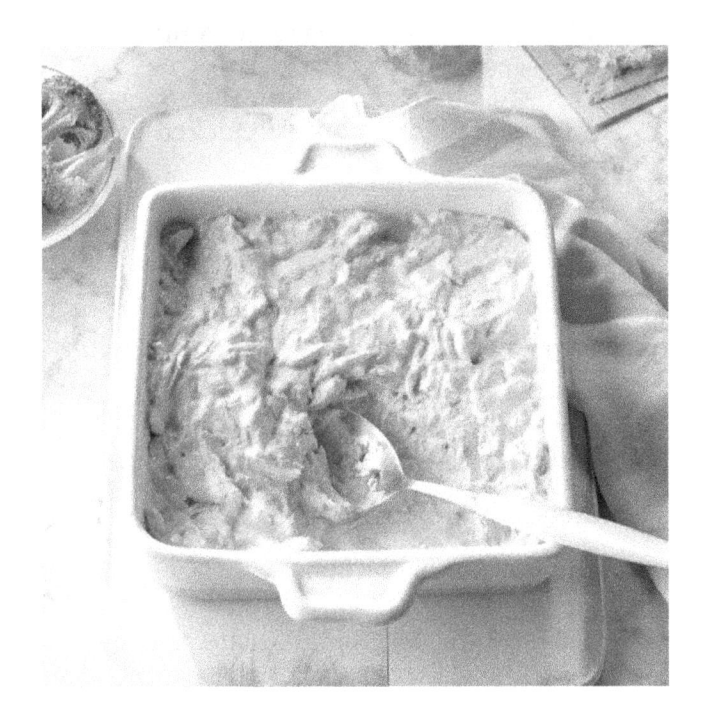

Prep/Total Time: 30 min.
Carbs per meal: 1g

Ingredients

1. 1 package (8 ounces) reduced-fat cream cheese

2. **1 cup reduced-fat sour cream**

3. **1/2 cup Louisiana-style hot sauce**

4. **3 cups shredded cooked chicken breast**

5. **Assorted crackers**

INSTRUCTIONS

- Preheat oven to 350°. In a large bowl, beat cream cheese, sour cream and hot sauce until smooth; stir in chicken.

- Transfer to an 8-in. square baking dish coated with cooking spray. Cover and bake until heated through, 18-22 minutes. Serve warm with crackers.

Better Than Fried Shrimp

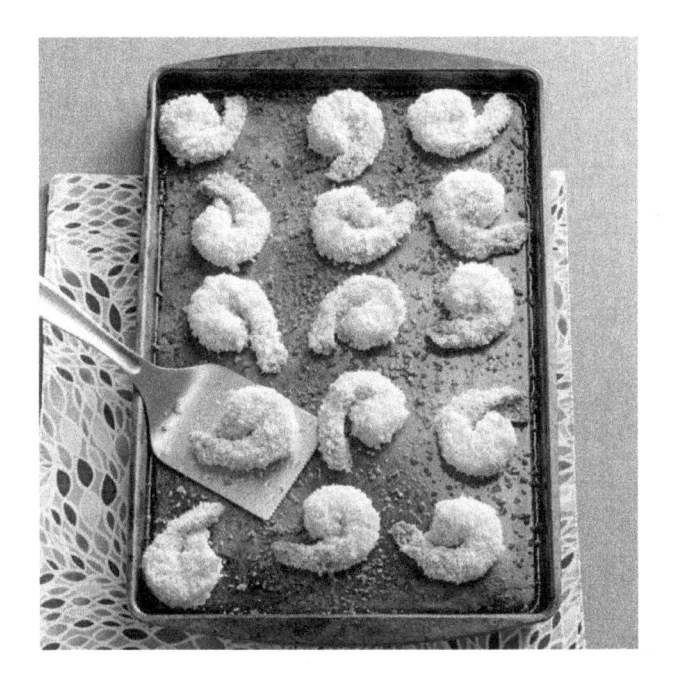

Prep/Total Time: 30 min.
Carbs per meal: 2g

Ingredients

1. 1-1/2 cups panko (Japanese) bread crumbs
2. 2 large egg whites
3. 1 tablespoon fat-free milk

4. 3 tablespoons all-purpose flour
5. 3 teaspoons seafood seasoning
6. 1/4 teaspoon salt
7. 1/4 teaspoon pepper
8. 30 uncooked large shrimp, peeled and deveined
9. Olive oil-flavored cooking spray

INSTRUCTIONS:

- Place bread crumbs in a shallow bowl. In another shallow bowl, combine egg whites and milk. In a third shallow bowl, combine flour, seafood seasoning, salt and pepper. Dip shrimp in the flour mixture, egg mixture, then bread crumbs.

- Place shrimp on a baking sheet coated with cooking spray; spritz shrimp with cooking spray. Bake at 400° for 8-12 minutes or until shrimp turn pink and coating is golden brown, turning once.

Walnut-Crusted Salmon

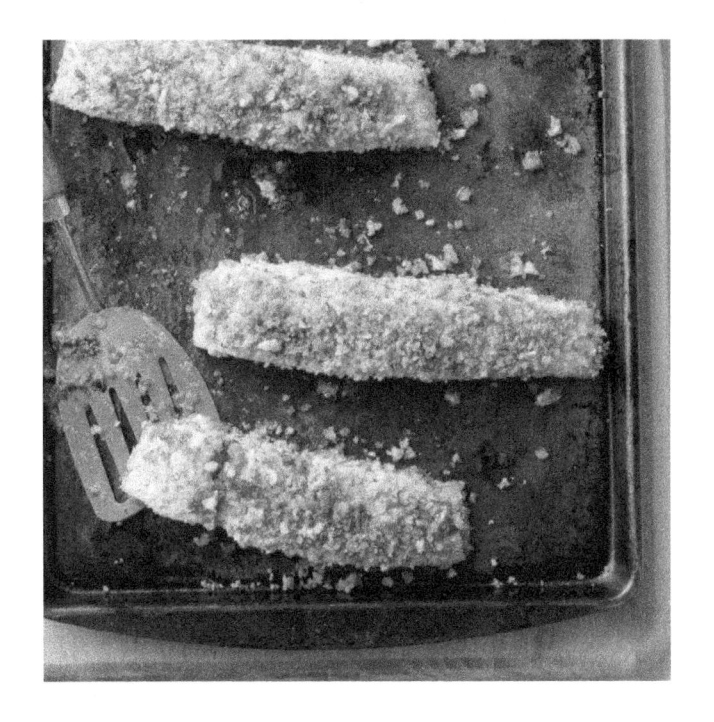

*Prep/Total Time: 25 min.
Carbs per meal: 13g*

Ingredients

1. 4 salmon fillets (4 ounces each)
2. 4 teaspoons Dijon mustard

3. 4 teaspoons honey

4. 2 slices whole wheat bread, torn into pieces

5. 3 tablespoons finely chopped walnuts

6. 2 teaspoons canola oil

7. 1/2 teaspoon dried thyme

INSTRUCTIONS:

- Preheat oven to 400°. Place salmon on a baking sheet coated with cooking spray. Mix mustard and honey; brush over salmon. Place bread in a food processor; pulse until coarse crumbs form. Transfer to a small bowl. Stir in walnuts, oil and thyme; press onto salmon.

- Bake 12-15 minutes or until topping is lightly browned and fish just begins to flake easily with a fork.

Grilled Honey-Lime Chicken

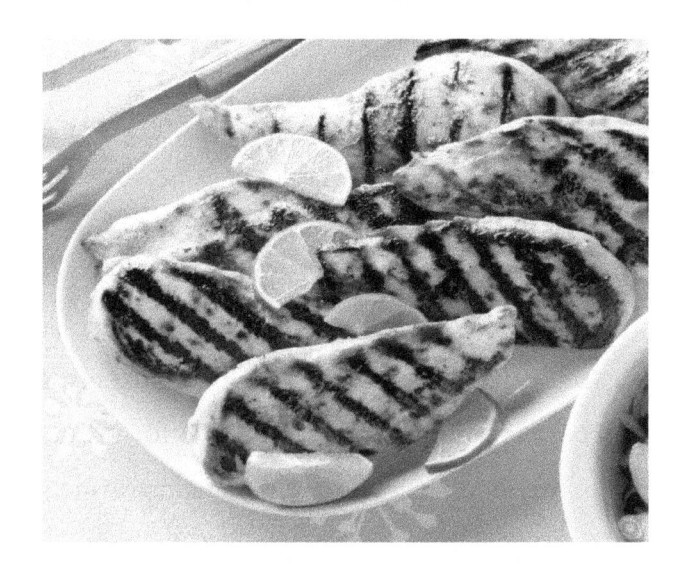

Prep: 10 min. + marinating Grill: 10 min.
Carbs per meal: 15g

Ingredients

1. 3/4 cup oil and vinegar salad dressing
2. 1/2 cup honey
3. 3 tablespoons lime juice
4. 1/2 teaspoon salt

5. 1/2 teaspoon pepper

6. 8 boneless skinless chicken breast halves (6 ounces each)

INSTRUCTIONS:

- In a small bowl, combine the first five ingredients. Pour 1 cup marinade into a large resealable plastic bag; add the chicken. Seal bag and turn to coat; refrigerate for 2 hours. Cover and refrigerate remaining marinade.

- Drain and discard marinade. Lightly oil the grill rack. Grill chicken, covered, over medium heat or broil 4 in. from the heat for 4-5 minutes on each side, or until a thermometer reads 170°, basting occasionally with reserved marinade.

Honey Grilled Shrimp

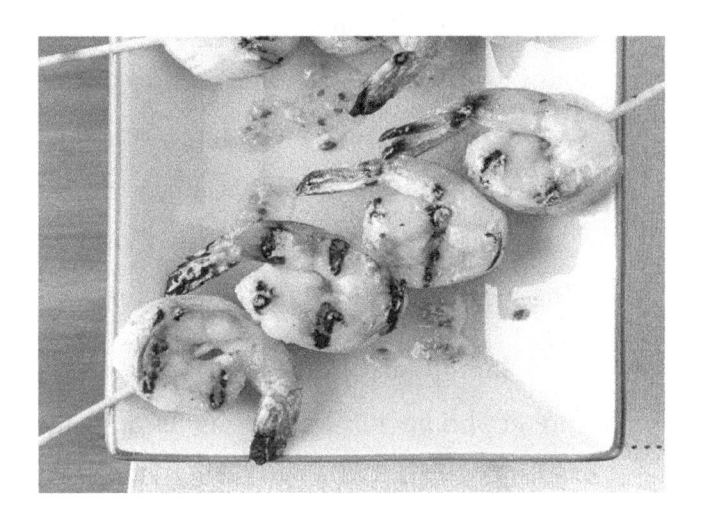

Prep: 20 min. + marinating Grill: 10 min.
Carbs per meal: 14g

Ingredients

1. 3/4 cup Italian salad dressing
2. 3/4 cup honey
3. 1/4 teaspoon minced garlic
4. 2 pounds uncooked medium shrimp, peeled and deveined

INSTRUCTIONS:

- In a small bowl, combine the salad dressing, honey and garlic; set aside 1/2 cup. Pour remaining marinade into a large resealable plastic bag; add the shrimp. Seal bag and turn to coat; refrigerate for 30 minutes. Cover and refrigerate reserved marinade for basting.

- Drain shrimp, discarding marinade from bag. Thread shrimp onto eight metal or soaked wooden skewers. On a greased grill rack, grill, uncovered, over medium heat or broil 4 in. from the heat for 1-1/2 to 2 minutes on each side. Baste with reserved marinade. Grill or broil 2-3 minutes longer or until shrimp are pink and firm, turning and basting frequently.

Corn with Cilantro-Lime Butter

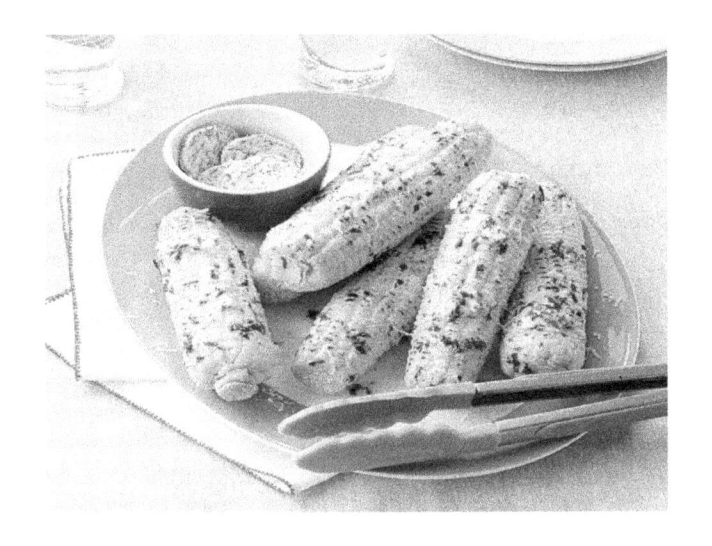

*Prep: 15 min. + chilling Grill: 15 min.
Carbs per meal: 17g*

Ingredients

1. 1/2 cup butter, softened
2. 1/4 cup minced fresh cilantro
3. 1 tablespoon lime juice
4. 1-1/2 teaspoons grated lime zest
5. 12 medium ears sweet corn, husks removed

6. Grated cotija cheese, optional

INSTRUCTIONS:

- In a small bowl, mix butter, cilantro, lime juice and lime zest. Shape into a log; wrap in plastic. Refrigerate 30 minutes or until firm. Wrap each ear of corn with a piece of heavy-duty foil (about 14 in. square).

- Grill corn, covered, over medium heat 15-20 minutes or until tender, turning occasionally. Meanwhile, cut lime butter into 12 slices. Remove corn from grill. Carefully open foil, allowing steam to escape. Serve corn with butter and, if desired, cheese.

Grilled Huli Huli Chicken

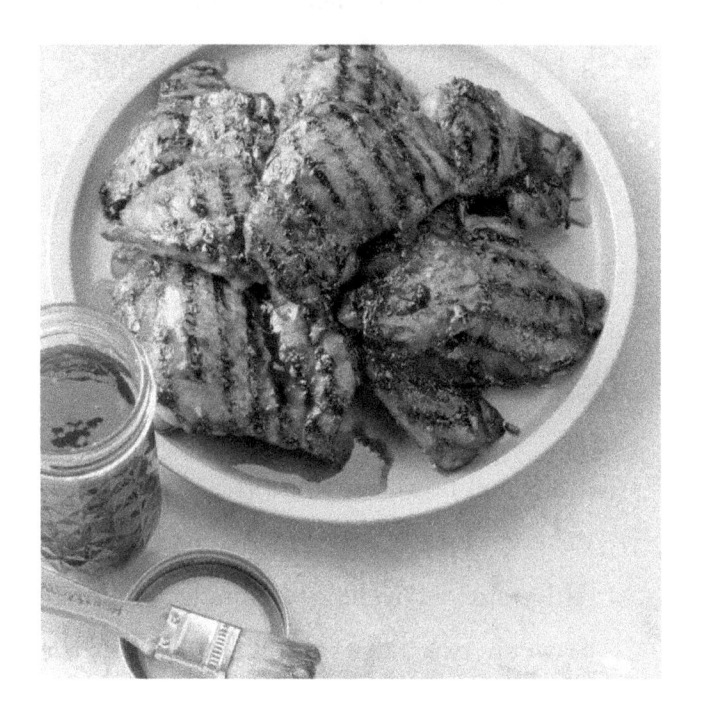

Prep: 15 min. + marinating Grill: 15 min
Carbs per meal: 15g

Ingredients

1. 1 cup packed brown sugar
2. 3/4 cup ketchup

3. 3/4 cup reduced-sodium soy sauce
4. 1/3 cup sherry or chicken broth
5. 2-1/2 teaspoons minced fresh gingerroot
6. 1-1/2 teaspoons minced garlic
7. 24 boneless skinless chicken thighs (about 5 pounds)

INSTRUCTIONS:

- In a small bowl, mix the first six ingredients. Reserve 1-1/3 cups for basting; cover and refrigerate. Divide remaining marinade between two large resealable plastic bags. Add 12 chicken thighs to each; seal bags and turn to coat. Refrigerate for 8 hours or overnight.
- Drain and discard marinade from chicken.
- Grill chicken, covered, on an oiled rack over medium heat for 6-8 minutes on each side or until no longer pink; baste occasionally with reserved marinade during the last 5 minutes.

Test Kitchen Tips

- For grilling, we love the moistness of chicken thighs, and they're economical, too. But use any cut of chicken you like.
- This sweet and savory glaze is also fantastic on pork chops.
- Transport yourself to Hawaii without firing up the grill! Pat chicken dry with paper towels; sear in a touch of oil in a skillet or grill pan. Transfer to a 375-degree oven for basting and baking.

Grilled Vegetable Platter

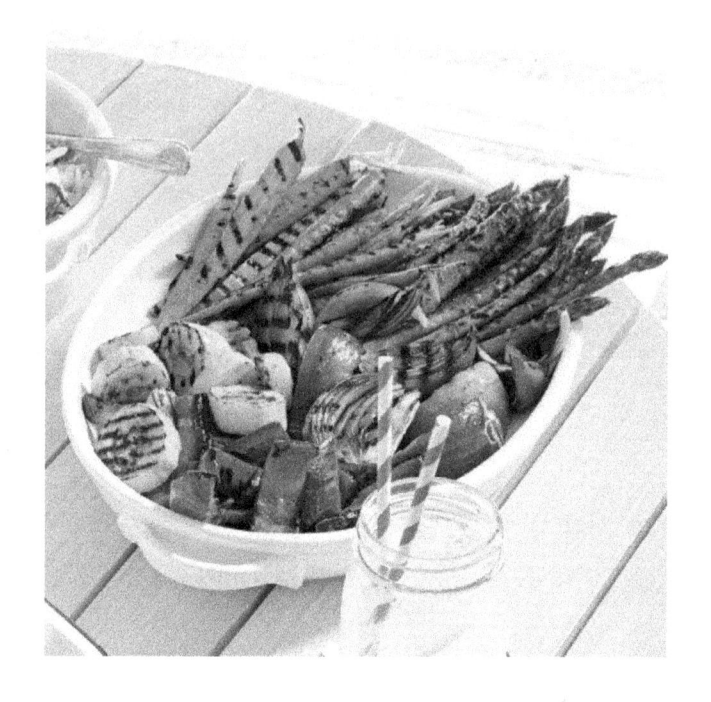

Prep: 20 min. + marinating Grill: 10 min
Carbs per meal: 15g

Ingredients

1. 1/4 cup olive oil
2. 2 tablespoons honey

3. 4 teaspoons balsamic vinegar

4. 1 teaspoon dried oregano

5. 1/2 teaspoon garlic powder

6. 1/8 teaspoon pepper

7. Dash salt

8. 1 pound fresh asparagus, trimmed

9. 3 small carrots, cut in half lengthwise

10. 1 large sweet red pepper, cut into 1-inch strips

11. 1 medium yellow summer squash, cut into 1/2-inch slices

12. 1 medium red onion, cut into wedges

INSTRUCTIONS:

- In a small bowl, whisk the first seven ingredients. Place 3 tablespoons marinade in a large resealable plastic bag. Add vegetables; seal bag and turn to coat. Marinate 1-1/2 hours at room temperature.

- Transfer vegetables to a grilling grid; place grid on grill rack. Grill vegetables, covered, over medium heat 8-12 minutes or until crisp-tender, turning occasionally.
- Place vegetables on a large serving plate. Drizzle with remaining marinade.

Editor's Note: If you do not have a grilling grid, use a disposable foil pan. Poke holes in the bottom of the pan with a meat fork to allow liquid to drain.

Contest-Winning Grilled Mushrooms

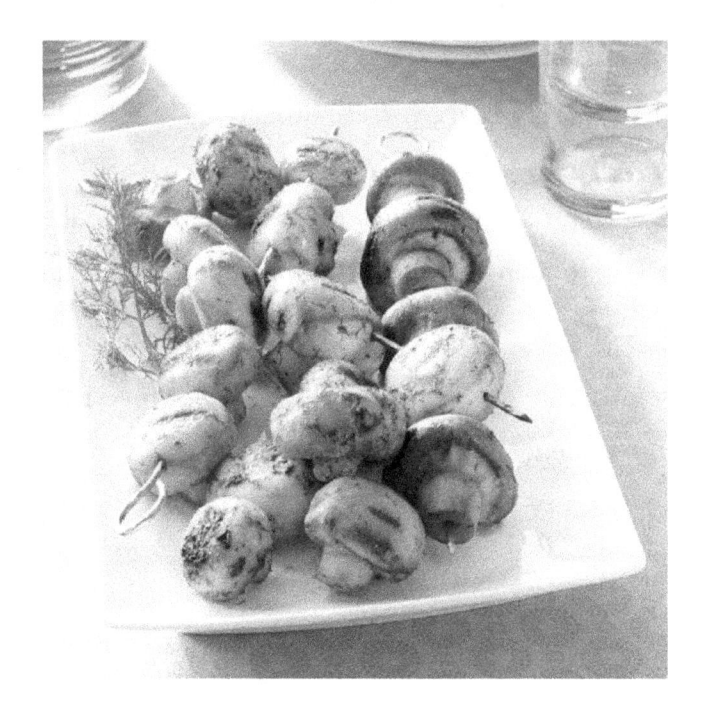

Prep/Total Time: 15 min.
Carbs per meal: 8g

INGREDIENTS:

1. 1/2 pound medium fresh mushrooms
2. 1/4 cup butter, melted

3. 1/2 teaspoon dill weed

4. 1/2 teaspoon garlic salt

INSTRUCTIONS:

- Thread mushrooms on four metal or soaked wooden skewers. Combine butter, dill and garlic salt; brush over mushrooms.
- Grill over medium-high heat for 10-15 minutes or until tender, basting and turning every 5 minutes.

30-Minute Chicken Noodle Soup

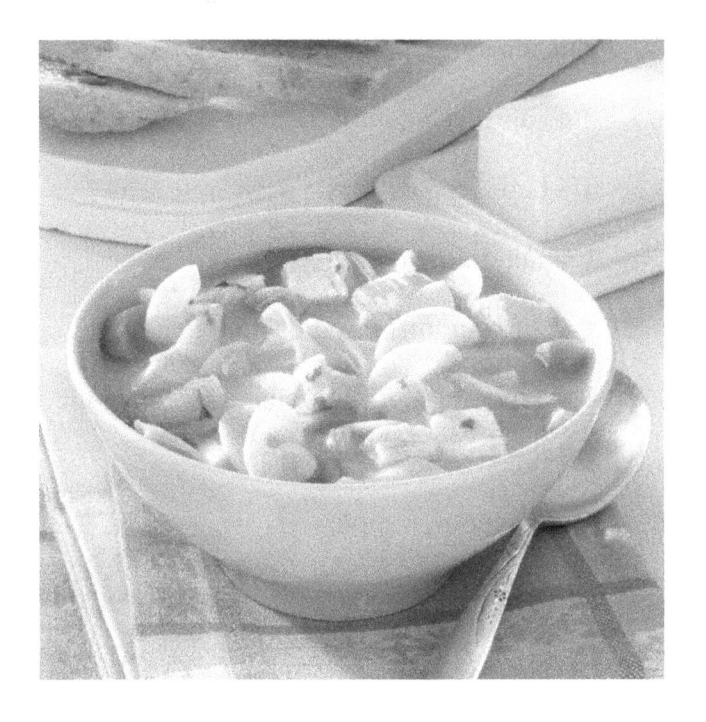

Prep/Total Time: 30 min.
Carbs per meal: 22g

Ingredients

1. 4 cups water
2. 1 can (14-1/2 ounces) chicken broth

3. 1-1/2 cups cubed cooked chicken breast
4. 1 can (10-3/4 ounces) condensed cream of chicken soup, undiluted
5. 3/4 cup sliced celery
6. 3/4 cup sliced carrots
7. 1 small onion, chopped
8. 1-1/2 teaspoons dried parsley flakes
9. 1 teaspoon reduced-sodium chicken bouillon granules
10. 1/4 teaspoon pepper
11. 3 cups uncooked egg noodles

INSTRUCTIONS:

- In a Dutch oven, combine the first 10 ingredients. Bring to a boil. Reduce heat; cover and simmer for 10 minutes or until vegetables are crisp-tender. Stir in noodles; cook 5-7 minutes longer or until noodles and vegetables are tender.

Grilled Fajitas

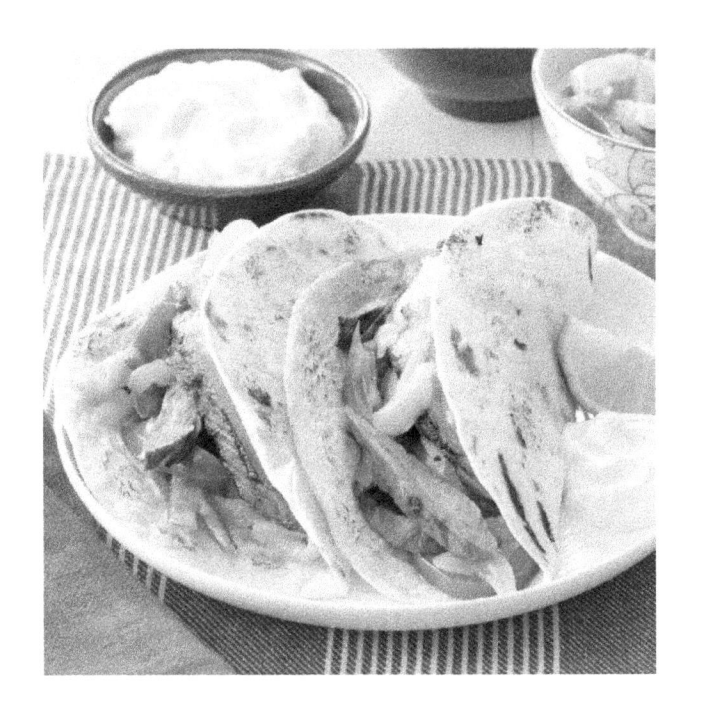

*Prep: 20 min. + marinating Grill: 10 min.
Carbs per meal: 59g*

Ingredients

1. 1 beef flank steak (about 1 pound)

2. 1 envelope onion soup mix

3. 1/4 cup canola oil

4. 1/4 cup lime juice

5. 1/4 cup water

6. 2 garlic cloves, minced

7. 1 teaspoon grated lime zest

8. 1 teaspoon ground cumin

9. 1/2 teaspoon dried oregano

10. 1/4 teaspoon pepper

11. 1 medium onion, thinly sliced

12. Green, sweet red and/or yellow peppers, julienned

13. 1 tablespoon canola oil

14. 8 flour tortillas (8 inches), warmed

15. Sour cream and lime wedges, optional

INSTRUCTIONS:

- In a large shallow dish, combine the first nine ingredients; add steak. Turn to coat; cover and refrigerate 4 hours or overnight.

- Drain and discard marinade. Grill over high heat until meat reaches desired doneness (for medium-rare, a thermometer should read 135°; medium, 140°; medium-well, 145°).

- Meanwhile, in a small skillet, saute onion and peppers if desired in oil for 3-4 minutes or until crisp-tender. Slice meat into thin strips across the grain; place on tortillas. Top with vegetables; roll up. Serve with sour cream and lime wedges if desired.

Grilled Potato Skins

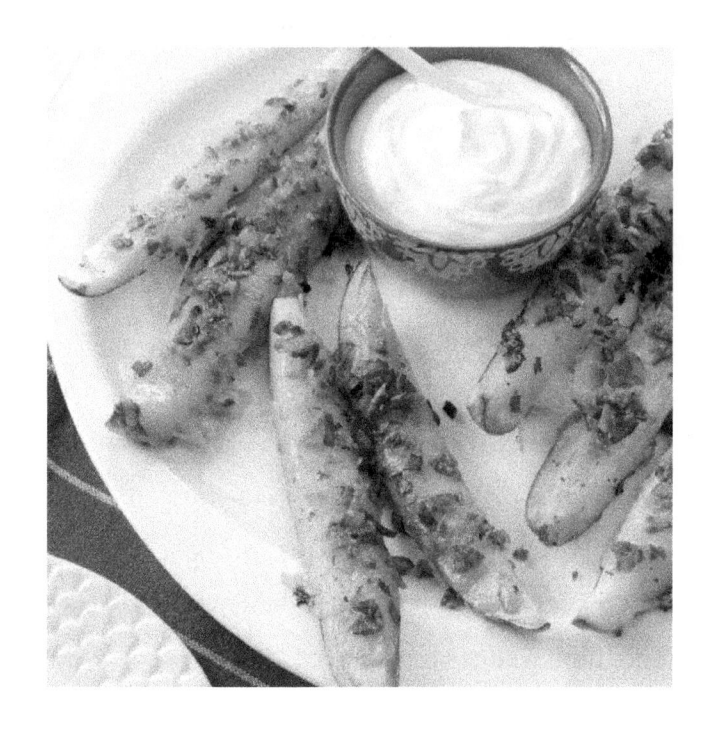

Prep/Total Time: 30 min.
Carbs per meal: 35g

Ingredients

1. 2 large baking potatoes
2. 2 tablespoons butter, melted

3. 2 teaspoons minced fresh rosemary or 1/2 teaspoon dried rosemary, crushed

4. 1/2 teaspoon salt

5. 1/2 teaspoon pepper

6. 1 cup shredded cheddar cheese

7. 3 bacon strips, cooked and crumbled

8. 2 green onions, chopped

9. Sour cream

INSTRUCTIONS:

- Cut each potato lengthwise into four wedges. Cut away the white portion, leaving 1/4 in. on the potato skins. Place skins on a microwave-safe plate. Microwave, uncovered, on high for 8-10 minutes or until tender. Combine the butter, rosemary, salt and pepper; brush over both sides of potato skins.

- Grill potatoes, skin side up, uncovered, over direct medium heat for 2-3 minutes or until lightly browned. Turn potatoes and position over indirect heat; grill 2 minutes longer. Top with cheese. Cover and grill 2-3 minutes longer or until cheese is melted. Sprinkle with bacon and onions. Serve with sour cream.

Rice on the Grill

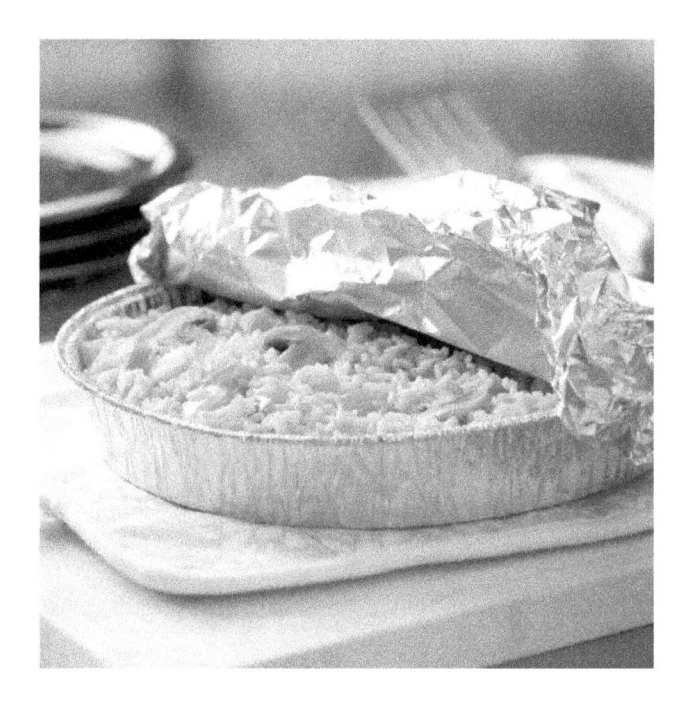

Prep/Total Time: 30 min.
Carbs per meal: 21g

Ingredients

1. 1-1/3 cups uncooked instant rice
2. 1/3 cup sliced fresh mushrooms

3. 1/4 cup chopped green pepper
4. 1/4 cup chopped onion
5. 1/2 cup water
6. 1/2 cup chicken broth
7. 1/3 cup ketchup
8. 1 tablespoon butter

INSTRUCTIONS:

- In a 9-in. round disposable foil pan, combine the first seven ingredients. Dot with butter. Cover with heavy-duty foil; seal edges tightly.

- Grill, covered, over medium heat for 12-15 minutes or until liquid is absorbed. Remove foil carefully to allow steam to escape. Fluff with a fork.

Balsamic-Glazed Beef Skewers

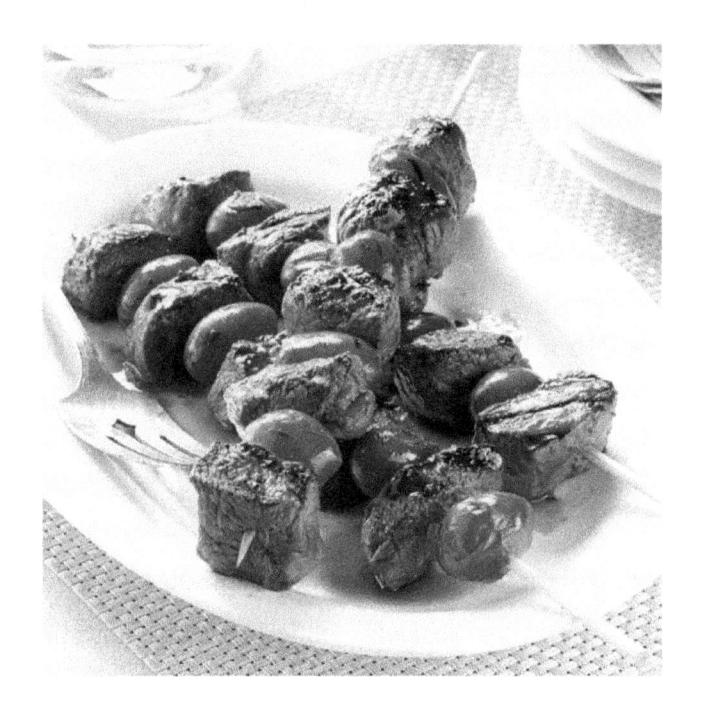

Prep/Total Time: 25 min.
Carbs per meal: 7g

Ingredients

1. 1/4 cup balsamic vinaigrette
2. 1/4 cup barbecue sauce

3. 1 teaspoon Dijon mustard
4. 1 pound beef top sirloin steak, cut into 1-inch cubes
5. 2 cups cherry tomatoes

INSTRUCTIONS:

- In a large bowl, whisk vinaigrette, barbecue sauce and mustard until blended. Reserve 1/4 cup mixture for basting. Add beef to remaining mixture; toss to coat.
- Alternately thread beef and tomatoes on four metal or soaked wooden skewers. Lightly grease grill rack.
- Grill skewers, covered, over medium heat or broil 4 in. from heat 6-9 minutes or until beef reaches desired doneness, turning occasionally and basting frequently with reserved vinaigrette mixture during the last 3 minutes.

Hot Quick Banana Boats

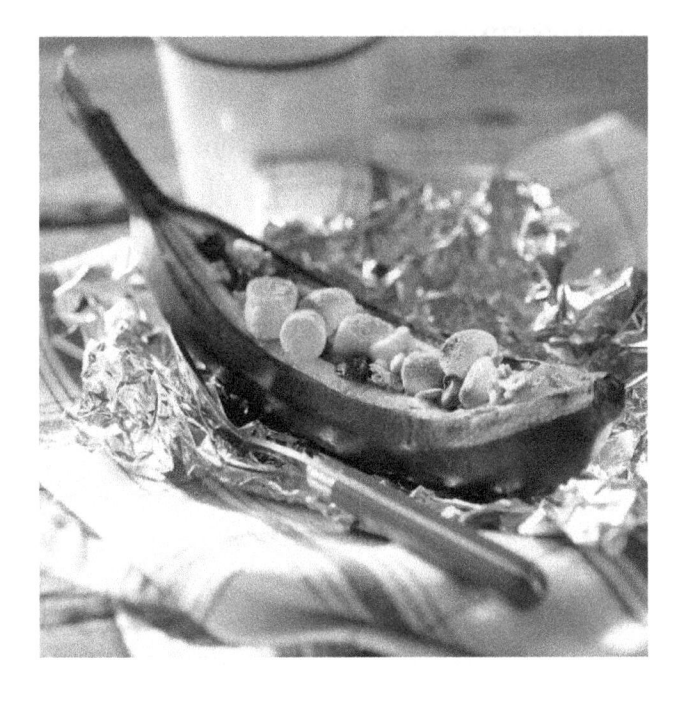

Prep/Total Time: 20 min.
Carbs per meal: 41g

Ingredients

1. 4 large unpeeled bananas
2. 8 teaspoons semisweet chocolate chips
3. 8 teaspoons trail mix

4. 1/4 cup miniature marshmallows

INSTRUCTIONS:

- Place each banana on a 12-in. square of foil; crimp and shape foil around bananas so they sit flat. Do not close over top.

- Cut each banana lengthwise about 1/2 in. deep, leaving 1/2 in. uncut at both ends. Gently pull each banana peel open, forming a pocket. Fill pockets with chocolate chips, trail mix and marshmallows.

- Grill bananas, covered, over medium heat for 4-5 minutes or until marshmallows are melted and golden brown.

Spinach and Mushroom Smothered Chicken

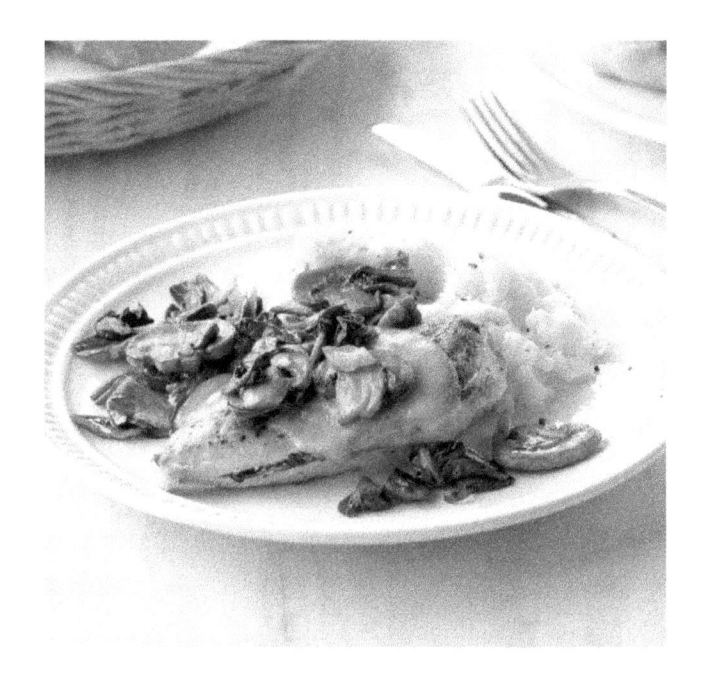

Prep/Total Time: 30 min.
Carbs per meal: 3g

Ingredients

1. 1-1/2 teaspoons olive oil
2. 1-3/4 cups sliced fresh mushrooms

3. 3 green onions, sliced

4. 3 cups fresh baby spinach

5. 2 tablespoons chopped pecans

6. 4 boneless skinless chicken breast halves (4 ounces each)

7. 1/2 teaspoon rotisserie chicken seasoning

8. 2 slices reduced-fat provolone cheese, halved

INSTRUCTIONS:

- Preheat grill or broiler. In a large skillet, heat oil over medium-high heat; saute mushrooms and green onions until tender. Stir in spinach and pecans until spinach is wilted. Remove from heat; keep warm.

- Sprinkle chicken with seasoning. Grill, covered, on an oiled grill rack over medium heat or broil 4 in. from heat on a greased broiler pan until a thermometer reads 165°, 4-5 minutes per side. Top with cheese; grill or broil until cheese is melted. To serve, top with mushroom mixture.

Health Tip: This low-carb main dish is also gluten-free.

Mushroom Cheese Bread

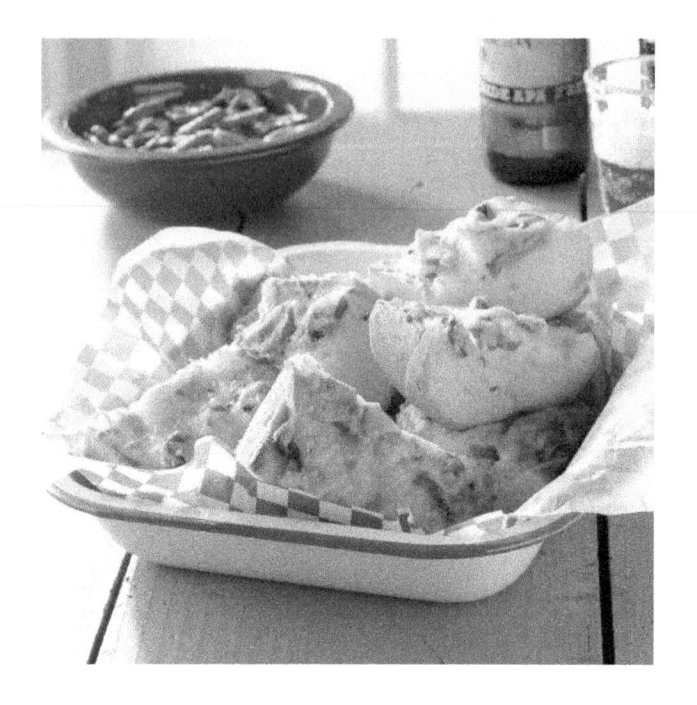

*Prep/Total Time: 15 min.
Carbs per meal: 20g*

Ingredients

1. 1 cup shredded part-skim mozzarella cheese
2. 1 can (4 ounces) mushroom stems and pieces, drained

3. 1/3 cup mayonnaise

4. 2 tablespoons shredded Parmesan cheese

5. 2 tablespoons chopped green onion

6. 1 loaf (1 pound) unsliced French bread

INSTRUCTIONS:

- In a small bowl, combine the mozzarella cheese, mushrooms, mayonnaise, Parmesan cheese and onion. Cut bread in half lengthwise; spread cheese mixture over cut sides.

- Grill, covered, over indirect heat or broil 4 in. from the heat until lightly browned, 5-10 minutes. Slice and serve warm.

Grilled Tilapia Piccata

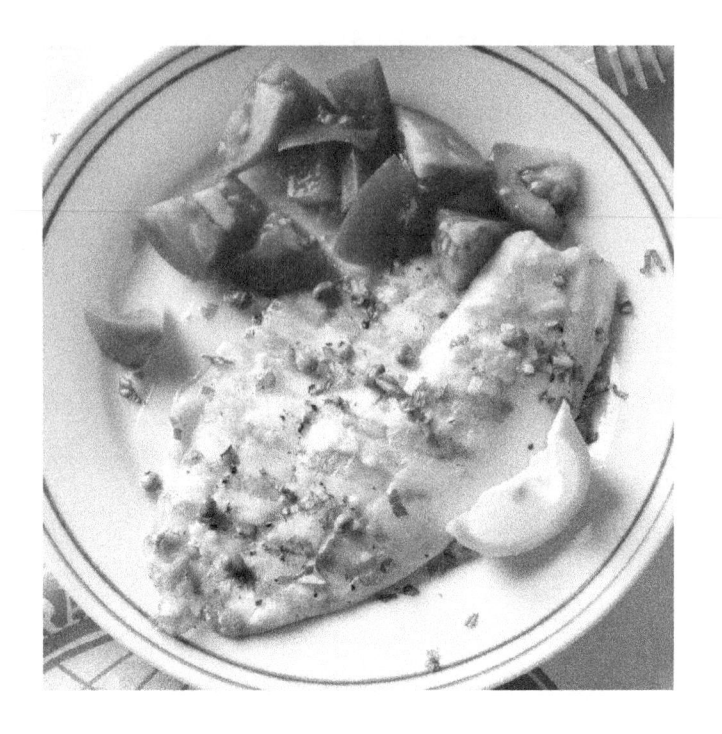

Prep/Total Time: 25 min
Carbs per meal: 2g

Ingredients

1. 1/2 teaspoon grated lemon zest

2. 3 tablespoons lemon juice

3. 2 tablespoons olive oil
4. 2 garlic cloves, minced
5. 2 teaspoons capers, drained
6. 3 tablespoons minced fresh basil, divided
7. 4 tilapia fillets (6 ounces each)
8. 1/2 teaspoon salt
9. 1/4 teaspoon pepper

INSTRUCTIONS:

- In a small bowl, whisk lemon zest, lemon juice, oil and garlic until blended; stir in capers and 2 tablespoons basil. Reserve 2 tablespoons mixture for drizzling cooked fish. Brush remaining mixture onto both sides of tilapia; sprinkle with salt and pepper.

- On a lightly oiled grill rack, grill tilapia, covered, over medium heat or broil 4 in. from heat 3-4 minutes on each side or until fish just begins to flake easily with a fork. Drizzle with reserved lemon mixture; sprinkle with remaining basil.

Health Tip: Look for U.S. or Canadian tilapia that's been farmed in closed tanks for the least impact on the environment.

Bruschetta from the Grill

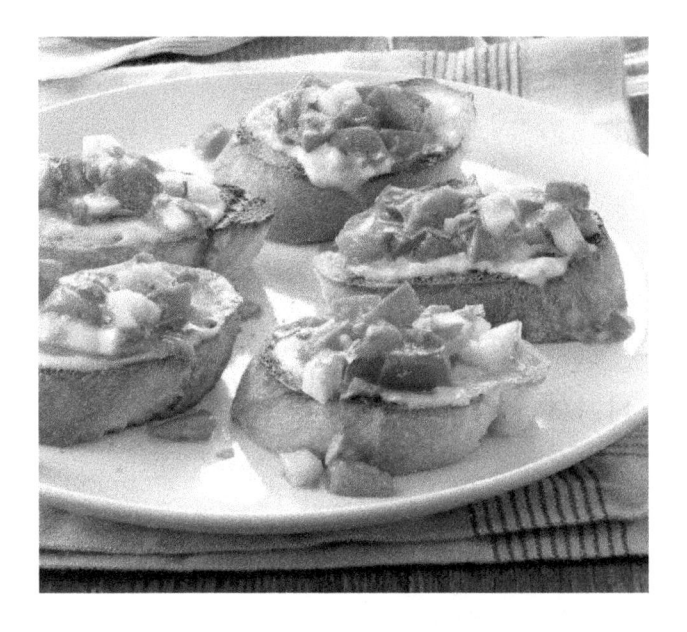

*Prep: 15 min. + chilling Grill: 5 min.
Carbs per meal: 28g*

Ingredients

1. 1 pound plum tomatoes (about 6), seeded and chopped
2. 1 cup chopped celery or fennel bulb
3. 1/4 cup minced fresh basil

4. 3 tablespoons balsamic vinegar

5. 3 tablespoons olive oil

6. 3 tablespoons Dijon mustard

7. 2 garlic cloves, minced

8. 1/2 teaspoon salt

9. MAYONNAISE SPREAD:

10. 1/2 cup mayonnaise

11. 1/4 cup Dijon mustard

12. 1 tablespoon finely chopped green onion

13. 1 garlic clove, minced

14. 3/4 teaspoon dried oregano

15. 1 loaf (1 pound) French bread, cut into 1/2-inch slices

INSTRUCTIONS:

- In a large bowl, combine the first eight ingredients. Cover and refrigerate for at least 30 minutes. For mayonnaise spread, in a small bowl, combine the mayonnaise, mustard, onion, garlic and oregano; set aside.

- Grill bread slices, uncovered, over medium-low heat for 1-2 minutes or until lightly toasted. Turn bread; spread with mayonnaise mixture. Grill 1-2 minutes longer or until bottoms of bread is toasted. Drain tomato mixture; spoon over tops.

Ultimate Grilled Pork Chops

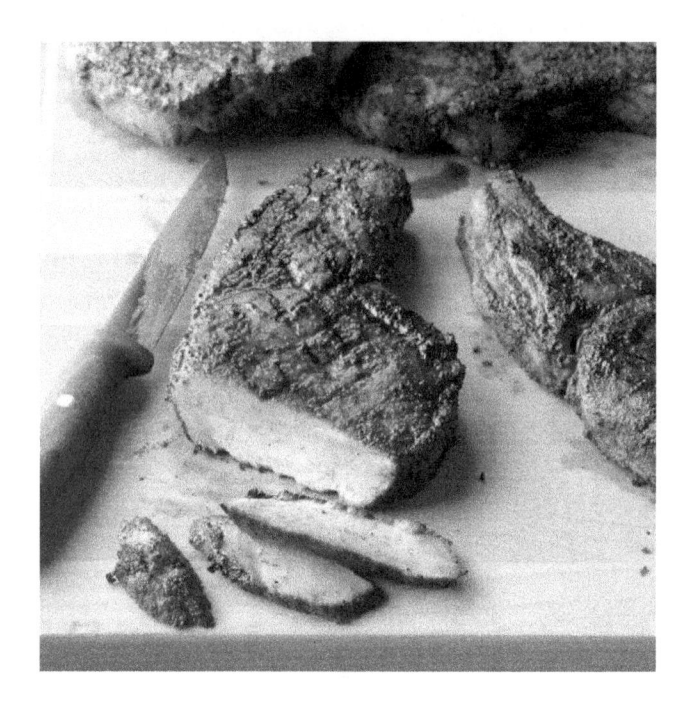

Prep: 20 min. + brining Grill: 10 min.
Carbs per meal: 5g

Ingredients

1. 1/4 cup kosher salt
2. 1/4 cup sugar

3. 2 cups water

4. 2 cups ice water

5. 4 center-cut pork rib chops (1 inch thick and 8 ounces each)

6. 2 tablespoons canola oil

7. BASIC RUB:

8. 3 tablespoons paprika

9. 1 teaspoon each garlic powder, onion powder, ground cumin and ground mustard

10. 1 teaspoon coarsely ground pepper

11. 1/2 teaspoon ground chipotle pepper

INSTRUCTIONS:

- In a large saucepan, combine salt, sugar and 2 cups water; cook and stir over medium heat until salt and sugar are dissolved. Remove from heat. Add 2 cups ice water to cool brine to room temperature.

- Place pork chops in a large resealable plastic bag; add cooled brine. Seal bag, pressing out as much air as possible; turn to coat chops. Place in a 13x9-in. baking dish. Refrigerate 8-12 hours.

- Remove chops from brine; rinse and pat dry. Discard brine. Brush both sides of chops with oil. In a small bowl, mix rub ingredients; rub over pork chops. Let stand at room temperature 30 minutes.

- Grill chops on an oiled rack, covered, over medium heat 4-6 minutes on each side or until a thermometer reads 145°. Let stand 5 minutes before serving.

Blue Cheese & Bacon Stuffed Peppers

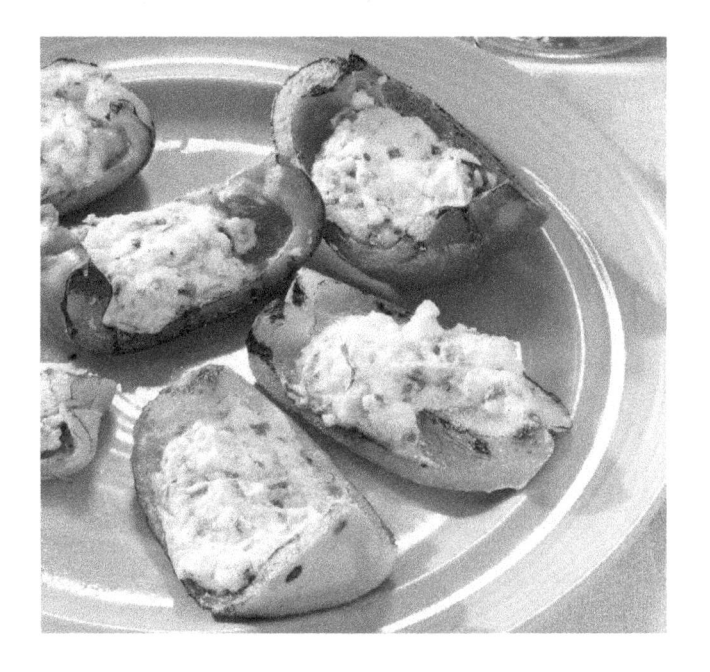

Prep/Total Time: 20 min.
Carbs per meal: 3g

Ingredients

1. 3 medium sweet yellow, orange or red peppers
2. 4 ounces cream cheese, softened

3. 1/2 cup crumbled blue cheese

4. 3 bacon strips, cooked and crumbled

5. 1 green onion, thinly sliced

INSTRUCTIONS:

- Cut peppers into quarters. Remove and discard stems and seeds. In a small bowl, mix cream cheese, blue cheese, bacon and green onion until blended.

- Grill peppers, covered, over medium-high heat or broil 4 in. from heat until slightly charred, 2-3 minutes on each side.

- Remove peppers from grill; fill each with about 1 tablespoon cheese mixture. Grill until cheese is melted, 2-3 minutes longer.

Summer Steak Kabobs

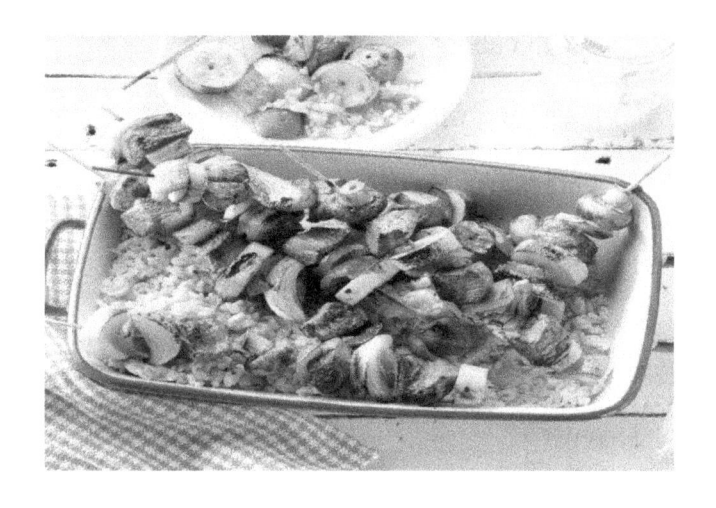

*Prep: 20 min. + marinating Grill: 10 min.
Carbs per meal: 11g*

Ingredients

1. 1/2 cup canola oil
2. 1/4 cup soy sauce
3. 3 tablespoons honey
4. 2 tablespoons white vinegar
5. 1/2 teaspoon ground ginger

6. 1/2 teaspoon garlic powder

7. 1-1/2 pounds beef top sirloin steak, cut into 1-inch cubes

8. 1/2 pound whole fresh mushrooms

9. 2 medium onions, cut into wedges

10. 1 medium sweet red pepper, cut into 1-inch pieces

11. 1 medium green pepper, cut into 1-inch pieces

12. 1 medium yellow summer squash, cut into 1/2-inch slices

13. Hot cooked rice

INSTRUCTIONS:

- In a large bowl, combine first six ingredients. Add beef; turn to coat. Cover and refrigerate 8 hours or overnight.

- On 12 metal or soaked wooden skewers, alternately thread beef and vegetables; discard marinade. Grill kabobs, covered, over medium heat until beef reaches desired doneness, 10-12 minutes, turning occasionally. Serve with rice.

Grilled Potatoes with Bacon-Ranch Sauce

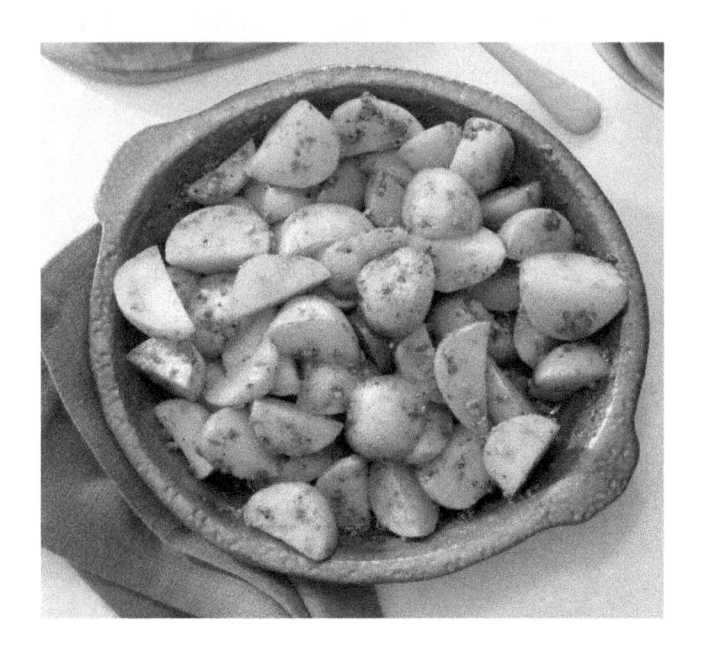

Prep/Total Time: 30 min.
Carbs per meal: 37g

Ingredients

1. 2 tablespoons olive oil
2. 1 tablespoon barbecue seasoning
3. 2 garlic cloves, minced

4. 2 teaspoons lemon juice
5. 1-1/2 pounds small potatoes, quartered
6. SAUCE:
7. 2/3 cup ranch salad dressing
8. 4 teaspoons bacon bits
9. 2 teaspoons minced chives
10. Dash hot pepper sauce

INSTRUCTIONS:

- In a large bowl, combine oil, barbecue seasoning, garlic and lemon juice. Add potatoes; toss to coat. Place on a double thickness of heavy-duty foil (about 28 in. square). Fold foil around potato mixture and seal tightly.
- Grill, covered, over medium heat 20-25 minutes or until potatoes are tender.
- In a small bowl, combine sauce ingredients. Serve with potatoes.

Flank Steak with Cilantro & Blue Cheese Butter

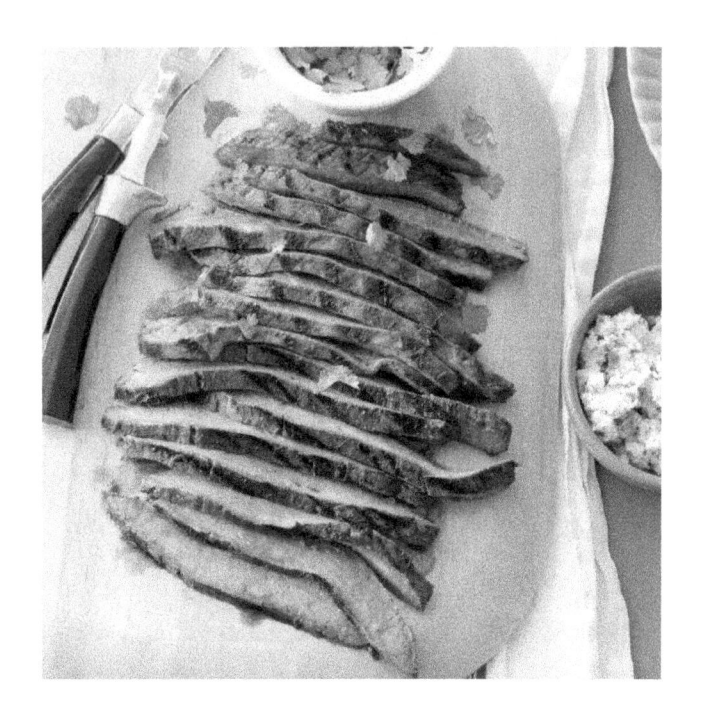

Prep: 15 min. + marinating Grill: 15 min.
Carbs per meal:3g

Ingredients

1. 1/2 cup canola oil
2. 1/4 cup cider vinegar

3. 1/4 cup honey

4. 1 tablespoon reduced-sodium soy sauce

5. 1/2 teaspoon paprika

6. 1 beef flank steak (2 pounds)

7. BLUE CHEESE BUTTER:

8. 3/4 cup crumbled blue cheese

9. 3 tablespoons butter, softened

10. 1 green onion, finely chopped

11. 1 tablespoon minced fresh cilantro

12. 1/8 teaspoon salt

13. 1/8 teaspoon pepper

INSTRUCTIONS:

- In a shallow dish, combine the first five ingredients. Add steak; turn to coat. Cover and refrigerate 2-4 hours.

- Drain beef, discarding marinade. Grill steak, covered, over medium heat or broil 4 in. from heat 6-8 minutes on each side or until meat reaches desired doneness (for medium-rare, a thermometer should read 135°; medium, 140°; medium-well, 145°). Let steak stand 5 minutes before thinly slicing across the grain.

- In a small bowl, beat blue cheese butter ingredients until blended. Serve steak with butter.

Grilled Jalapenos

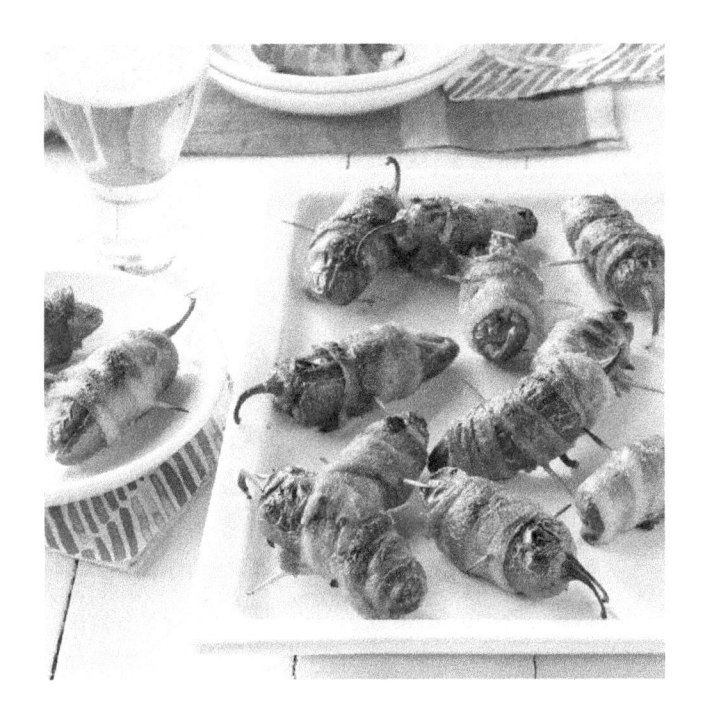

Prep/Total Time: 25 min.
Carbs per meal: 1g

Ingredients

1. 24 fresh jalapeno peppers
2. 3/4 pound bulk pork sausage

3. 12 bacon strips, halved

INSTRUCTIONS:

- Wash peppers. Cut a slit along one side of each pepper. Remove seeds; rinse and dry peppers.

- In a skillet, cook sausage over medium heat until no longer pink; drain. Stuff peppers with sausage and wrap with bacon; secure with soaked toothpicks.

- Grill peppers, uncovered, turning frequently, over medium heat until tender and bacon is crisp, about 15 minutes.

Note

Wear disposable gloves when cutting hot peppers; the oils can burn skin. Avoid touching your face.

Grilled Pork Tenderloins

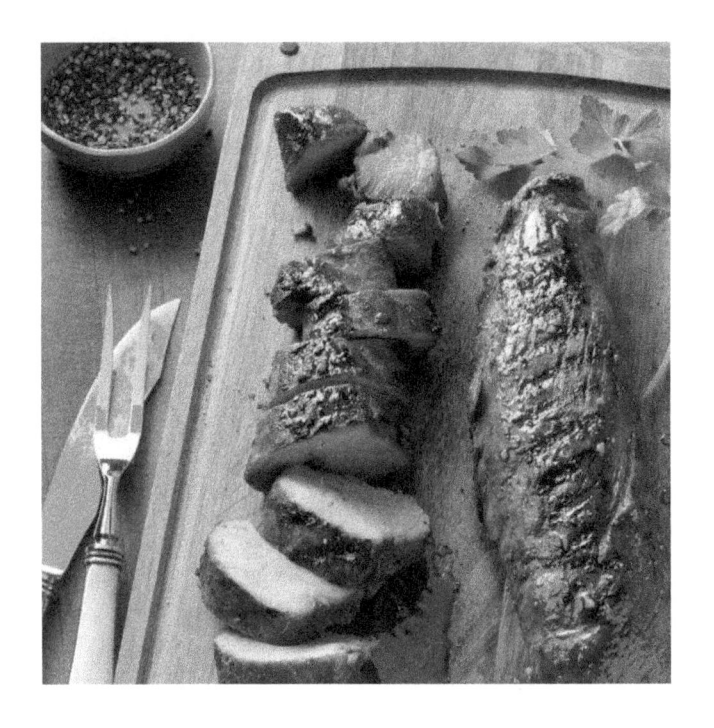

*Prep: 10 min. + marinating Grill: 20 min.
Carbs per meal: 15g*

Ingredients

1. 1/3 cup honey
2. 1/3 cup reduced-sodium soy sauce

3. 1/3 cup teriyaki sauce

4. 3 tablespoons brown sugar

5. 1 tablespoon minced fresh gingerroot

6. 3 garlic cloves, minced

7. 4 teaspoons ketchup

8. 1/2 teaspoon onion powder

9. 1/2 teaspoon ground cinnamon

10. 1/4 teaspoon cayenne pepper

11. 2 pork tenderloins (about 1 pound each)

12. Hot cooked rice

INSTRUCTIONS:

- In a large bowl, combine the first 10 ingredients. Pour half of the marinade into a large resealable plastic bag; add tenderloins. Seal bag and turn to coat; refrigerate 8 hours or overnight, turning occasionally. Cover and refrigerate remaining marinade.

- Drain and discard marinade from meat. Grill, covered, over indirect medium-hot heat for 20-35 minutes or until a thermometer reads 145°, turning occasionally and basting with reserved marinade. Let stand 5 minutes before slicing. Serve with rice.

- Freeze option: Freeze uncooked pork in bag with marinade. Transfer reserved marinade to a freezer container; freeze. To use, completely thaw tenderloins and marinade in refrigerator. Grill as directed.

Triple Tomato Flatbread

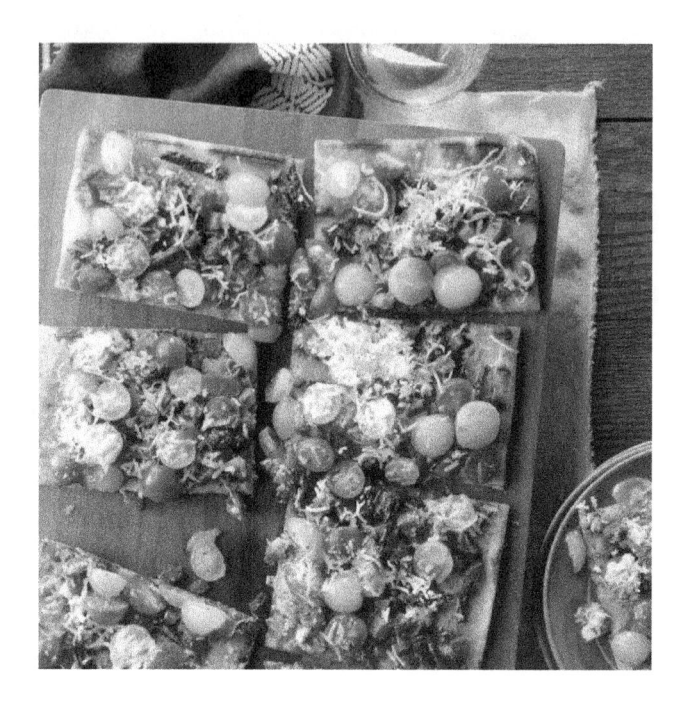

*Prep/Total Time: 20 min.
Carbs per meal: 29g*

Ingredients

1. 1 tube (13.8 ounces) refrigerated pizza crust
2. Cooking spray

3. 3 plum tomatoes, finely chopped (about 2 cups)
4. 1/2 cup soft sun-dried tomato halves (not packed in oil), julienned
5. 2 tablespoons olive oil
6. 1 tablespoon dried basil
7. 1/4 teaspoon salt
8. 1/4 teaspoon pepper
9. 1 cup shredded Asiago cheese
10. 2 cups yellow and/or red cherry tomatoes, halved

INSTRUCTIONS:

- Unroll and press dough into a 15x10-in. rectangle. Transfer dough to an 18x12-in. piece of heavy-duty foil coated with cooking spray; spritz dough with cooking spray. In a large bowl, toss plum tomatoes and sun-dried tomatoes with oil and seasonings.

- Carefully invert dough onto grill rack; remove foil. Grill, covered, over medium heat 2-3 minutes or until bottom is golden brown. Turn; grill 1-2 minutes longer or until second side begins to brown.

- Remove from grill. Spoon plum tomato mixture over crust; top with cheese and cherry tomatoes. Return flatbread to grill. Grill, covered, 2-4 minutes or until crust is golden brown and cheese is melted.

- To bake flatbread: Preheat oven to 425°. Unroll and press dough onto bottom of a 15x10x1-in. baking pan coated with cooking spray. Bake 6-8 minutes or until lightly browned. Assemble flatbread as directed. Bake 8-10 minutes longer or until crust is golden and cheese is melted.

Italian Sausage and Provolone Skewers

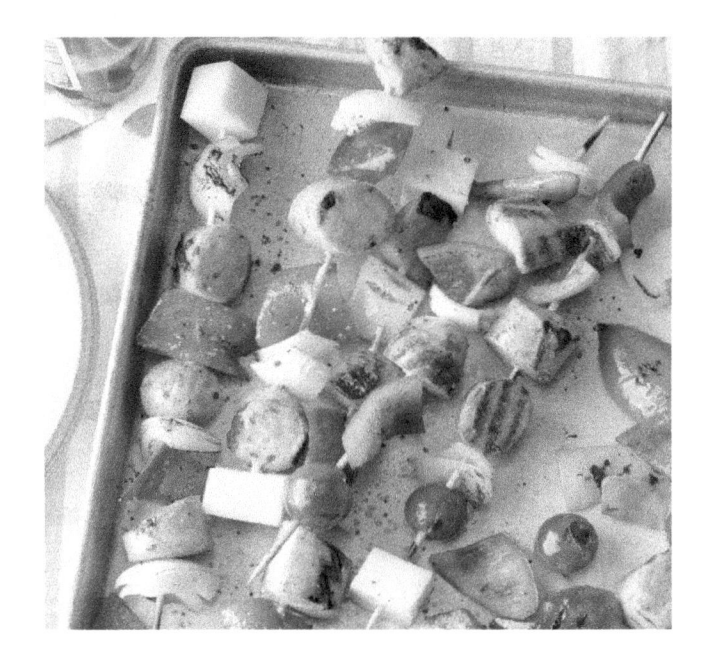

*Prep/Total Time: 30 min.
Carbs per meal: 7g*

Ingredients

1. 1 large onion
2. 1 large sweet red pepper
3. 1 large green pepper

4. 2 cups cherry tomatoes

5. 1 tablespoon olive oil

6. 1/2 teaspoon pepper

7. 1/4 teaspoon salt

8. 2 packages (12 ounces each) fully cooked Italian chicken sausage links, cut into 1-1/4-inch slices

9. 16 cubes provolone cheese (3/4 inch each)

INSTRUCTIONS:

- Cut onion and peppers into 1-in. pieces; place in a large bowl. Add tomatoes, oil, pepper and salt; toss to coat. On 16 metal or soaked wooden skewers, alternately thread sausage and vegetables.

- Grill, covered, over medium heat 8-10 minutes or until sausage is heated through and vegetables are tender, turning occasionally. Remove kabobs from grill; thread one cheese cube onto each kabob.

CHICKEN CAPRESE ZOODLE BOWLS

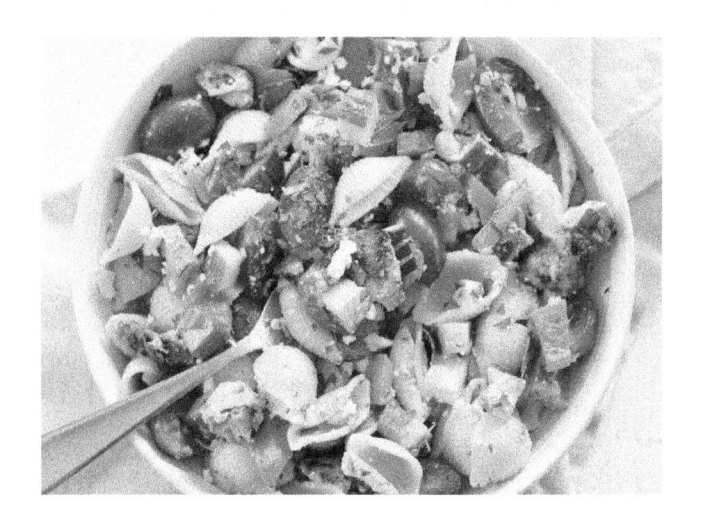

Prep time: 5 minutes
Cook time: 20 minutes
Carbs per meal: 22g

Ingredients

1. 1 lb boneless skinless chicken breast cleaned and pounded- thin 2 large zucchini

2. c cherry tomatoes halved

3. ½ c mini mozzarella balls halved

4. ¼ c chopped basil separated

5. tablespoons olive oil separated

6. 2 tablespoons balsamic vinegar for dressing

7. Sea salt + pepper

Instructions

- In a large skillet heat 1 tbsp olive oil. Cook chicken 7-8 minutes on each side until browned.

- Spiralize 2 large zucchini, Chop tomatoes, mozzarella, and basil.

- In a bowl combine zoodles, cherry tomatoes, mozzarella balls, basil, olive oil, salt + pepper. Toss until everything is thoroughly coated.

- Plate the zoodles and top with cooked chicken and balsamic glaze

LOW CARB PIZZA CHICKEN SKILLET

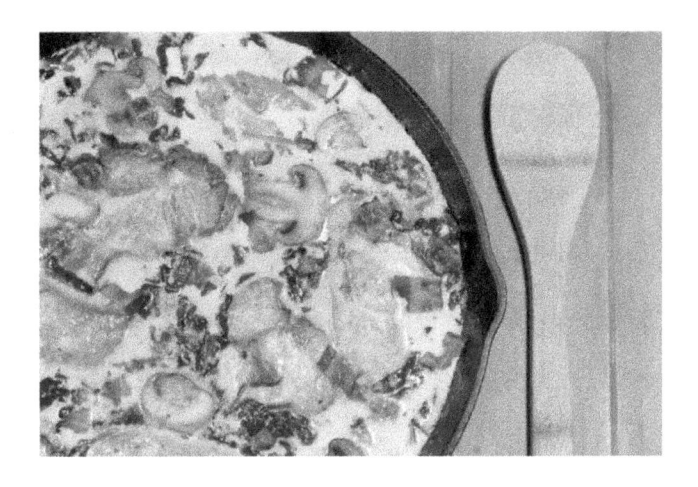

Aneasy low carb chicken skillet recipe that's so simple to prepare. Just brown boneless skinless chicken meat and smother with pizza toppings.

Prep time: 5 mins
Cook time: 15 mins
Carbs per meal: 21g

Ingredients

1. 2 tablespoons avocado oil or olive oil

1. 5 pounds skinless/boneless chicken pieces about 5 thighs
2. 1/4 teaspoon salt sprinkle to taste
3. 1/8 teaspoon pepper sprinkle to taste
4. 2 cloves garlic minced
5. 1 cup low carb pizza sauce or marinara sauce
6. 5 slices mozzarella cheese
7. 1 ounce pepperoni slices

Instructions

- Heat oil in skillet over medium high heat. Season chicken with salt and pepper.
- Add seasoned chicken and garlic to skillet. Cook chicken until browned.
- Pour pizza or marinara sauce on top. Allow to simmer until sauce is heated.
- Top each piece of chicken with a slice of mozzarella cheese and pieces of pepperoni.

- Cover skillet until cheese is melted or place skillet under broiler to melt cheese and serve immediately.

TEQUILA LIME CHICKEN

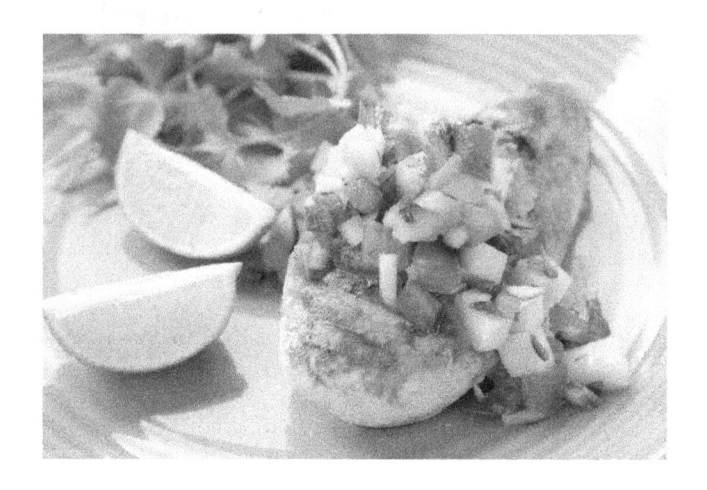

Tequila Lime Chicken is packed with vibrantflavors and cooks in under 30 min- A fun and festive Mexican-style dish perfect for friday night dinner parties and week-night meals alike!

Prep time: 15 mins
Cook time: 7 mins
Carbs per meal: 27g

Ingredients

1. 2 skinless free-range organic chicken breasts

2. 1 tbsp olive oil, for grilling For the marinade:

3. 1 tbsp extravirgin olive oil ¼ cup good-quality gold tequila zest of 2 limes

4. 1 tsp light honey

5. 1 tbsp hot or mild paprika powder

6. 1 thai red chilli, finely minced 1 garlic clove, finely minced a generous pinch of sea salt and cayenne pepper To serve:

7. ½ cup pinepple salsa lime wedges fresh cilantro, chopped

Instructions

- Whisk all the marinade ingredients together in a bowl. Add the chicken breasts into the marinade, and stir well to combine.

- Divide the chicken into two zip-log bags, and pour half the marinade on each breast. Close the bags and marinate in the fridge for 15 minutes but best for 2 hours.

- Drizzle with oil a grill pan, and heat until medium-high heat.

- Place the chicken breasts on the grill and spoon any remaining marinade from the bag over top. Grill, covered, for 4 minutes one one side. Turn the breast and cook a further 5 mins.

- Serve immediately with lime wedges on the side, and top with fresh cilantro and a spoonful of pineapple salsa

CHICKEN AND CAULIFLOWER SKILLET

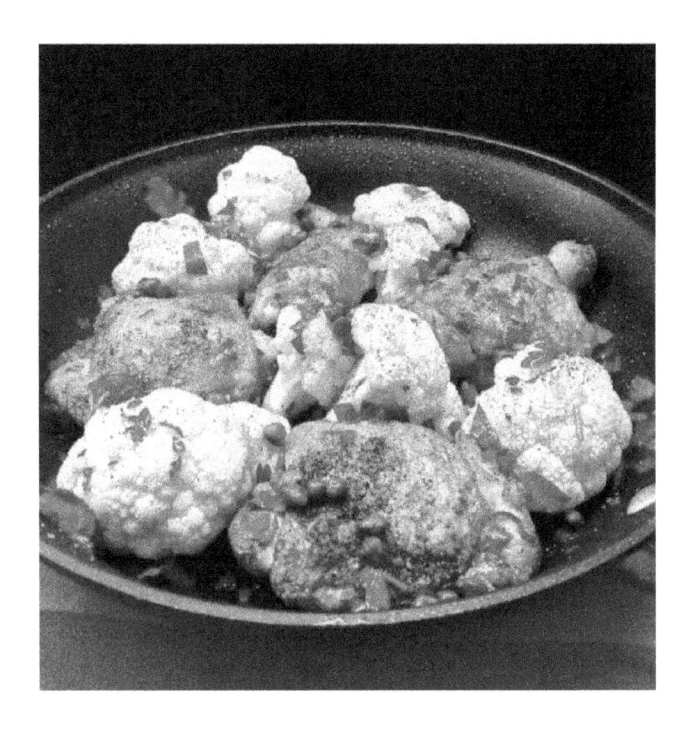

Healthy Chicken Cauliflower Skillet features sauteed chicken baked with yummy cauliflower, covered with a sherry vinegar sauce, parsley, and capers.

Prep time: 10 mins

Cook time: 30 mins
Carbs per meal: 14g

Ingredients

1. 4 chicken thighs bone-in, skin-on
2. 1 Tbsp olive oil
3. 1 head cauliflower broken up into large florets
4. 1/4 cup fresh parsley chopped
5. 3 Tbsp sherry vinegar
6. 2 Tbsp capers

Instructions

- Preheat your oven to 450 degrees.
- Heat a large oven-proof skillet over medium-high heat. Add the olive oil. Season the chicken thighs with salt and pepper, place in the skillet skin side down. Cook the chicken for 5-6 minutes, or until the skin is golden

brown. Turn the chicken over and cook for an additional 3-4 minutes.

- Remove from the heat, arrange the cauliflower florets around the chicken and make sure to coat them with the pan juices. Season lightly with salt and pepper.

- Put the skillet in the oven and cook for about 20 minutes, or until the chicken is done and the cauliflower is crisp-tender.

- Carefully remove the pan from the oven, add the sherry vinegar, and sprinkle the parsley and capers over the chicken. Serve immediately. Enjoy!

BROILED CHICKEN THIGHS WITH ARTICHOKES AND GARLIC

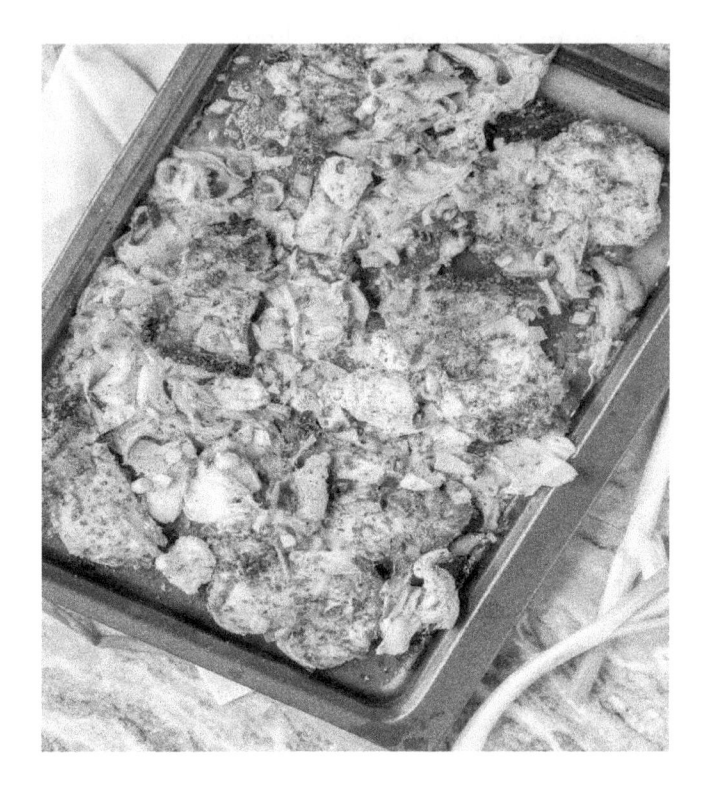

Only 4 key ingredients needed for these low fuss, minimal clean up 30 minute artichoke and garlic broiled chicken thighs. A classic go to weeknight dinner recipe. Healthy and delicious. Gluten Free and Dairy Free.

Prep time: 10 mins
Cook time: 20 mins - Carbs per meal: 29g

Ingredients

1. 1.5 pounds boneless skinless chicken thighs 6
2. 1-2 jars artichoke hearts (10 ounce jars)
3. tablespoons dried oregano 2 tablespoons minced garlic salt and pepper to taste

Instructions

- Mix chicken thighs and artichoke hearts (including liquid) in a large bowl. Allow to marinate for 20-30 minutes (optional).
- Drain the liquid.
- Add oregano, minced garlic, salt and pepper and mix.

- Broil on high for 20-25 minutes or until chicken is cooked through. (Broil on the second or third rack from the top for the first 20 minutes and then place the baking tray on the top oven shelf - closer to the broiler, to get a nice crisp on the chicken for the last 5 minutes)
- Optional: halfway through cooking time you can flip over the chicken thighs, if you like.

CUMIN SPICED BEEF WRAPS – LOW CARB, PALEO

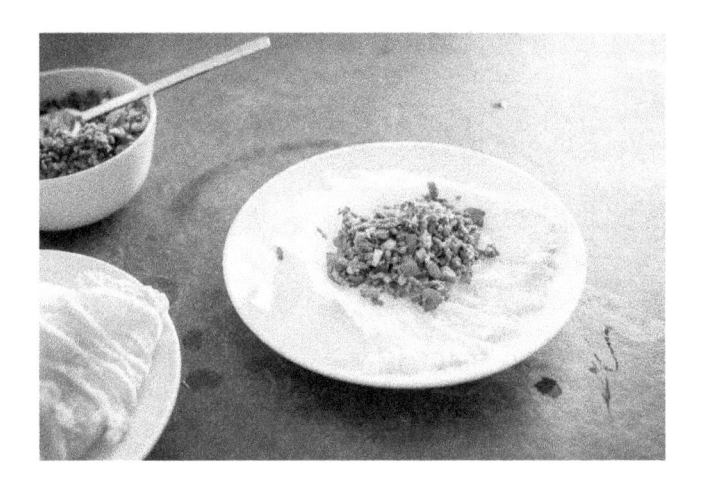

Prep time: 15 mins
Cook time: 10 mins
Carbs per meal: 9g

Ingredients

1. 1-2 tbsp coconut oil
2. 1/4 onion, diced small
3. 2/3 lb ground beef
4. red bell pepper, diced small

5. tbsp cilantro, chopped
6. 1 tsp ginger, minced
7. 4 cloves garlic, minced
8. 2 tsp cumin
9. Salt and pepper, to taste
10. 8 large cabbage leaves (savoy cabbage or Napa cabbage)

Instructions

- Place 1-2 tbsp of coconut oil into a frying pan and sauté the onions, ground beef, and peppers on medium heat.
- When the ground beef is cooked, add in the cilantro, ginger, garlic, cumin, salt, and pepper to taste.
-
- Fill a large pot 3/4 full with water and bring to a boil.

- Using tongs, blanch each cabbage leaf in the boiling water (put each leaf into the boiling water for 20 seconds). Then plunge each leaf into some cold water before draining and placing onto a plate.
- Spoon the beef mixture onto each lettuce leaf and fold into a roll.

LEMON AND THYME CHICKEN THIGHS

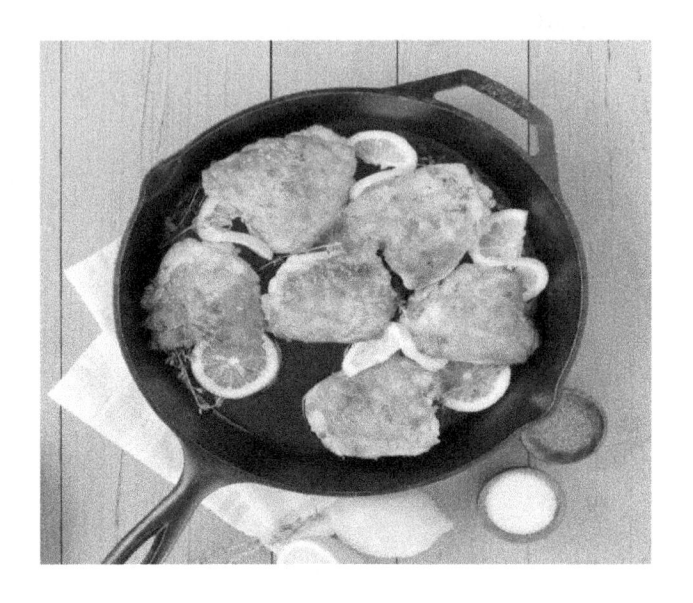

This recipe highlights how great high-quality chicken can taste when combined with just a little seasoning, fresh herbs and lemon juice. This combination allows the chicken to stay very moist, tender and full of nutrients. Ideal as a meal, snack or even as a picnic dish the following day.

Prep time: 5 mins
Cook time: 30 mins
Carbs per meal: 18g

Ingredients

1. 6 bone-in, skin-on chicken thighs (2 pounds)//
2. ½ teaspoon fine sea salt
3. ½ teaspoon ground black pepper
4. ½ teaspoon garlic powder
5. 1 tablespoon ghee, lard or tallow
6. 1 large lemon, sliced
7. 6 sprigs of fresh thyme
8. 1 tablespoon freshly squeezed lemon juice

Instructions

- Preheat the oven to 450°F.

- Sprinkle the chicken on both sides with the salt, pepper, and garlic powder.

- Heat the ghee in a large cast-iron skillet over medium-high heat.

- Place the chicken thighs in the pan, skin side down, and cook for 2 minutes.

- Reduce the heat to medium and continue cooking the thighs without touching them for another 10 minutes, or until the skin has released from the pan (the skin will initially stick to the pan and then will release once the fat has rendered).

- Drain any excess fat from the pan, then transfer the skillet to the oven (remember, the handle will be hot).

- Cook for 10 more minutes.

- Remove the skillet from the oven and flip the chicken pieces over.

- Nestle the lemon slices and thyme sprigs between the chicken pieces, then return the pan to the oven for 5 minutes, or until the skin is crispy and the juices run clear when a knife is inserted and the meat is no longer pink inside, or the internal temperature of the chicken reaches 165°F.

- Remove from the oven. Drizzle with lemon juice, and serve.

GRILLED CHICKEN, BACON & RADISHES

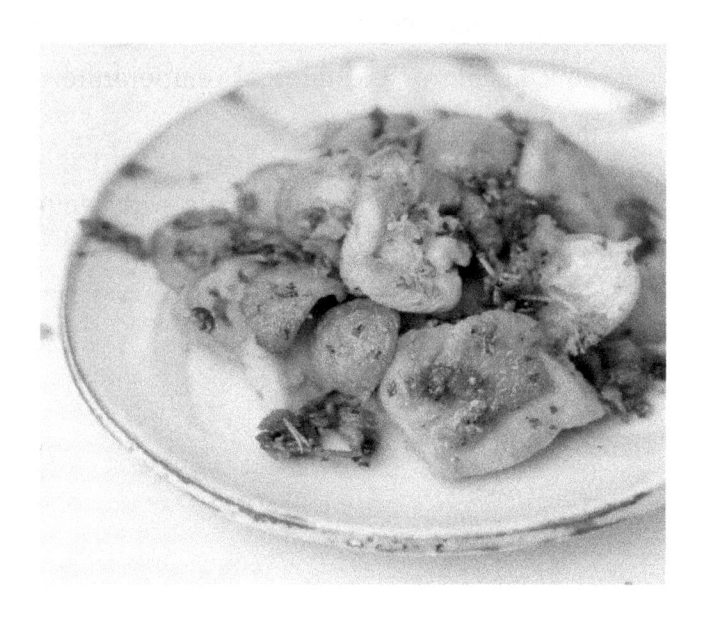

An easy dinner that everyone will love!

Prep time: 10 mins
Cook time: 10 mins
Carbs per meal: 15g

Ingredients

1. 10 slices bacon (about 150g raw)

2. 15 radishes (230g)

3. 2 boneless chicken thighs with skin (300g)

4. 2 cloves garlic

5. tsp extra virgin olive oil

6. 1/4 tsp Himalayan salt

7. 1/4 tsp black pepper

8. tsp rosemary

9. 2 tbsp chopped fresh parsley   pinch Himalayan salt pinch black pepper

INSTRUCTIONS

- Slice the radishes in half. Thinly slice the garlic. Cut the chicken into bite size pieces. Cut the bacon into 2cm strips. Sprinkle the 1/4 tsp of salt and pepper all over the chicken pieces.

- In a 10" cast iron skillet, heat the tsp of olive oil on medium heat and add the chicken pieces, skin side down. Grill for a minute so that they start to get a nice crisp, and add the bacon all around. Start frying for a few minutes and when the bacon is all cooked (not crispy), add the sliced radishes and garlic. Sprinkle the rosemary over everything and fry until the bacon is crispy, for 3-4 minutes. Sprinkle a bit of salt and pepper over everything and top with the chopped parsley.

PAN SEARED CHICKEN BREAST WITH MUSTARD CREAM SAUCE (LOW CARB, GLUTEN-FREE)

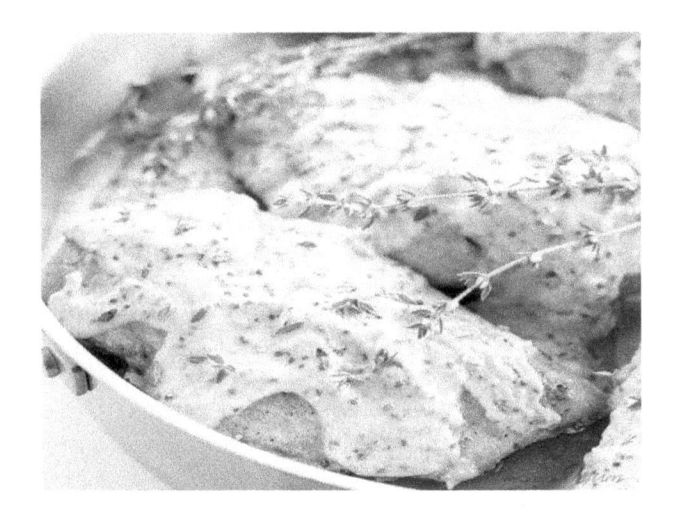

This quick & easy pan seared chicken breast recipe with mustard cream sauce takes just 15 minutes! It's the perfect healthy, flavorful weeknight dinner.

Cook time: 15 mins

Carbs per meal: 26g

Ingredients

1. 4 large Chicken breast
2. Sea salt
3. Black pepper
4. 2 tbsp Olive oil (divided)
5. 2 cloves Garlic (minced)
6. 1/2 cup Chicken broth
7. 2/3 cup Heavy cream (or coconut cream for paleo or whole 30)
8. tbsp Fresh thyme
9. tbsp Dijon mustard

Instructions

- Season the chicken breasts on both sides with sea salt and black pepper.

- Heat a tablespoon of oil in a pan over medium-high heat. Add the chicken and saute for 4-5 minutes on each side, until golden brown and cooked through.

- Transfer to a plate and cover to keep warm.

- Add the remaining tablespoon of oil to the pan, along with the garlic. Saute for about 30 seconds, until fragrant.

- Add the chicken broth. Stir to remove any bits stuck to the bottom of the pan. Simmer for a few minutes, until the liquid is reduced by half.

- Add the cream and thyme. (See notes for sweeter sauce.) Return to a gentle simmer. Gently simmer again for a couple of minutes, continuing to scrape any pieces from the bottom, just until the sauce thickens (it will reduce in volume).

- Stir in the mustard at the end and turn off heat.

- To serve, pour the sauce over the chicken, or transfer the chicken back to the pan and cover in sauce.

EASY PAN SEARED LAMB CHOPS WITH MUSTARD CREAM SAUCE

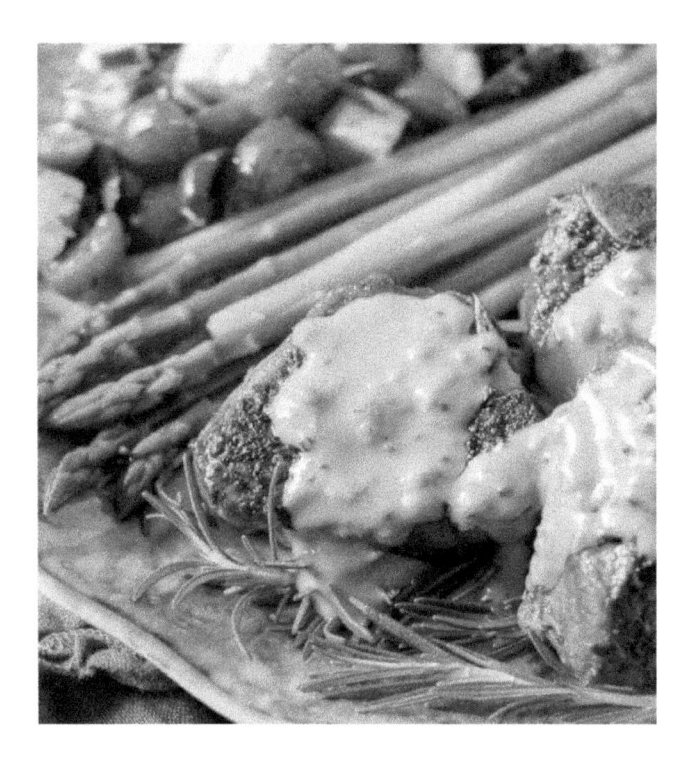

This easy pan seared lamb chop recipe flavors the lamb chops with a dry marinade of garlic and rosemary then finishes them with a silky, creamy, mustard pan sauce.

Prep time: 10 mins
Cook time: 20 mins
Carbs per meal: 18

Ingredients

PAN SEARED LAMB CHOPS

1. 1/2 pounds lamb chops, trimmed of excess fat, 6 chops
2. cloves garlic, minced
3. tablespoon rosemary, minced
4. tablespoons olive oil salt and pepper

MUSTARD CREAM PAN SAUCE

5. tablespoon shallot, minced
6. 1/2 cup beef broth, unsalted
7. tablespoons Brandy
8. 2/3 cup heavy cream
9. tablespoon grainy mustard like Maille

10. teaspoons lemon juice

11. 2 teaspoons Worcestershire sauce

12. teaspoon erythritol

13. sprig of rosemary and sprig of thyme

14. tablespoons butter salt and pepper to taste

Instructions

- Lamb Chop Prep: The day before - Place the minced rosemary and garlic in a small bowl with 1 tablespoon of olive oil. Trim off any excess fat (or stray bones) from the lamb chops, leaving a thin layer of fat about 1/8 of an inch. Place the lamb chops in a single layer in a shallow baking dish and season all sides with salt and pepper. Smear the garlic-rosemary-oil on both sides of each lamb chop. Cover with plastic wrap and refrigerate over-night.

- Prep: The day of - Bring the lamb to room temperature for 30 minutes. Mince the shallot and juice the lemon. Have the sprigs of rosemary and thyme ready. Put the other ingredients near the stove or have them measured and waiting. Cooking: Heat a large frying pan (non-stick or stainless) over medium high heat. When hot, add 1 tablespoon of oil, swirling to coat the pan. Add the lamb chops in one layer and turn heat down to medium. Let the lamb chops cook undisturbed for 6-7 minutes. Turn and cook again for another 6-7 minutes depending on how rare you like your lamb chops. Remove the lamb to a plate and cover loosely with foil.

- Mustard Cream Pan Sauce: Turn the heat down to medium-low and add the shallots, sauteing until softened. Add the beef broth and brandy and bring the heat back up to medium. Simmer for 1 minute and add the mustard, Worcestershire sauce and erythritol. Stir or whisk to combine.

- Whisk in the cream and add the sprig of rosemary and thyme. Let simmer for 7- 8 minutes or until almost your desired consistency - it will thicken as it cools. Add the lemon juice and butter, stir. Simmer until the sauce is glossy and thick. Check the seasoning.

- Remove the sprigs of rosemary and thyme before saucing the lamb chops and serving.

GREEK HERBED LAMB

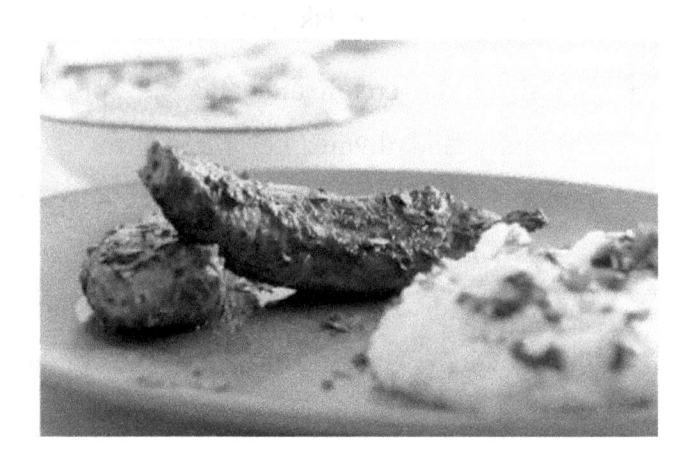

Greek Herbed Lamb is marinated in olive oil, lemon, garlic, oregano and parsley, giving it a fresh, spring taste. Your family will love this tasty, lowcarb, 30minute, Greek lamb recipe!

Prep time: 15 mins
Cook time: 15 mins
Carbs per meal: 33g

Ingredients

Lamb

1. 1.5 lb lamb tenderloin (fillet)
2. 1 tbsp extra virgin olive oil
3. lemon, juiced (2 tbsp)
4. 1/4 tsp pepper
5. tsp dried oregano
6. tsp dried parsley
7. 2-3 crushed garlic cloves

Cauliflower Mash

8. lb cauliflower chopped
9. 1 cup light single, pouring cream
10. 3 cups chicken broth
11. 1 oz unsalted butter chopped
12. Himalayan salt

Instructions

- Make mash: pour cream and chicken stock into a saucepan and turn on the heat.

- Break the florets off the cauliflower and chop roughly in half, add to the pan. Bring to the boil then lower the heat and simmer, covered for 15 mins.

- Once cauliflower is simmering, make the lamb marinade.

- Lamb marinade: Combine all the ingredients except the lamb in a small jug and mix to combine.

- Place lamb in a zip-lock bag and pour over the marinade. Close the bag and jiggle the lamb around so it's well coated. Leave to marinate for about 10 minutes.

- Place a fry-pan over medium-high heat and add 1 tbsp olive oil.

- Pan-fry the lamb for 3-4 minutes on each side. Rest for a few minutes if time permits.

- While the lamb is cooking, drain cauliflower which should be tender by now, reserving 1/4 cup of liquid.

- Use a food processor or immersion blender to blend the cauliflower, butter, salt and the reserved liquid until pureed.

- Serve the Mediterranean lamb with the cauliflower mash.

PERFECT BACON AND EGG CUPS

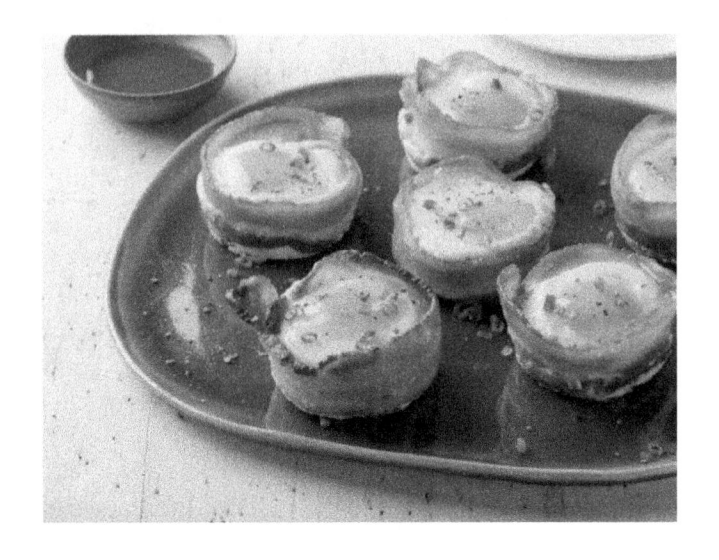

meal prep breakfast that is full of protein and portable.

Prep time: 10 mins
Cook time: 20 mins
Carbs per meal: 11g

Ingredients

1. 12 eggs

2. **12 pieces nitrate free bacon (paleo approved if necessary)**
3. **1 tbsp chopped chives salt and pepper**

Instructions

- Preheat oven to 400 degrees.
- Cook bacon for about 8-10 minutes. Remove from pan while still pliable, not crisp. Cool on paper towels.
- Grease your muffin tins.
- Put one piece of bacon in each hole, wrapping it around to line the sides. Crack the eggs in each hole. Top with chopped chives. Salt and pepper to taste.
- Cook for about 12-15 minutes or until bacon is crisp. Watch closely.

ROASTED BRUSSELS SPROUTS WITH BACON

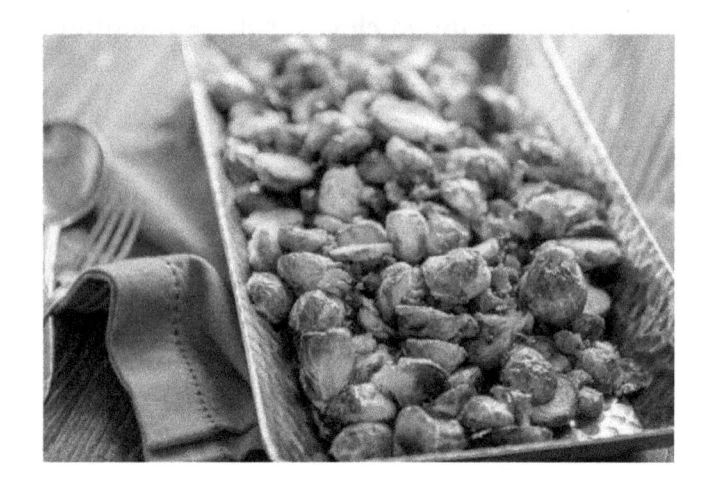

Prep time: 5 mins
Cook time: 25 mins
Carbs per meal: 23g

Ingredients

1. lb brussels sprouts

2. tbsp olive oil 8 strips bacon salt pepper

Instructions

- Preheat the oven to 375°F and cut the ends off of each brussels sprout, it's too tough. Then cut each in half, or even in quarters if they're very big.

- Throw them in a deep bowl and toss with olive oil, salt, pepper and any other spices you like. We sometimes toss them in red pepper and cumin!

- Pour them out onto a greased baking sheet making sure to leave a little bit a room between them. They don't all need to be on the same side, they'll all roast up nicely even if they look messy on that sheet.

- Place the baking sheet into the oven and bake for about 30 minutes. Halfway through, reach in to the oven and give the baking sheet a good shake so that the brussels sprouts rotate a little.

- While the brussels sprouts are baking, fry up as much bacon as you'd like. We use 2 pieces for each person we're feeding.

- When the bacon is cooked to your liking, chop it up into small pieces, roughly a half inch big, You want them bite sized.

- When the brussels sprouts have shriveled a bit and blackened, they're ready! Take them out of the oven and toss them in the same deep bowl with the bacon bits.

- Serve onto plates and give one last sprinkle of salt! Enjoy!

EASY TURKEY CHILI RECIPE

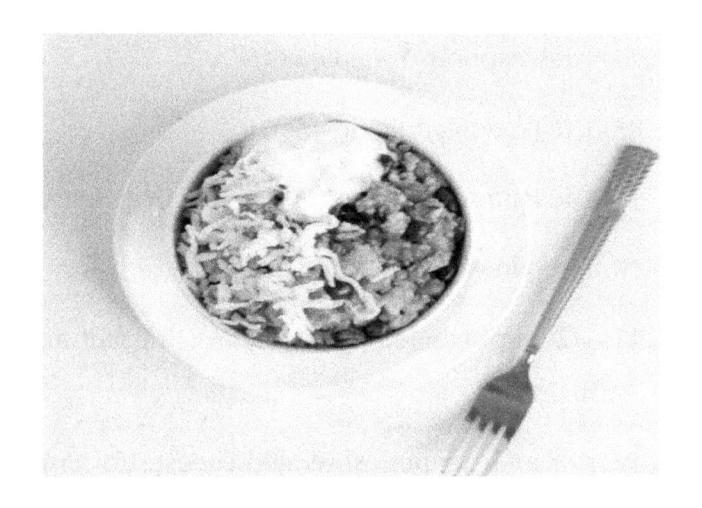

Prep time: 20 mins
Cook time: 10 mins
Carbs per meal: 24g

Ingredients

1. 1 tablespoon olive oil

2. 1 small yellow onion (diced)

3. small green pepper (diced)

4. cloves minced garlic

5. 2 pounds ground turkey breast (85% lean)
6. 1 1/2 tablespoons chili powder
7. 1 tablespoon ground cumin
8. 1 teaspoon garlic powder
9. 1 teaspoon cayenne (more if desired)
10. 1 cup low carb tomato sauce
11. 1/2 cup canned black beans (rinsed and drained)
12. salt and pepper shredded cheese (to serve) sour cream (to serve)

Instructions

- Heat the oil in a large skillet over medium-high heat.
- Add the onion and peppers then sauté for 2 to 3 minutes until browned.
- Stir in the garlic and cook for 1 minute more.
- Add the ground turkey and season with salt and pepper.

- Cook until the turkey is browned, breaking it up with a wooden spoon, then stir in the spices.

- Stir in the tomato sauce and black beans then simmer on medium-low for 10 minutes.

- Adjust the seasoning to taste then serve hot with shredded cheese and sour cream.

COUNTY FAIR CINNAMON DONUTS

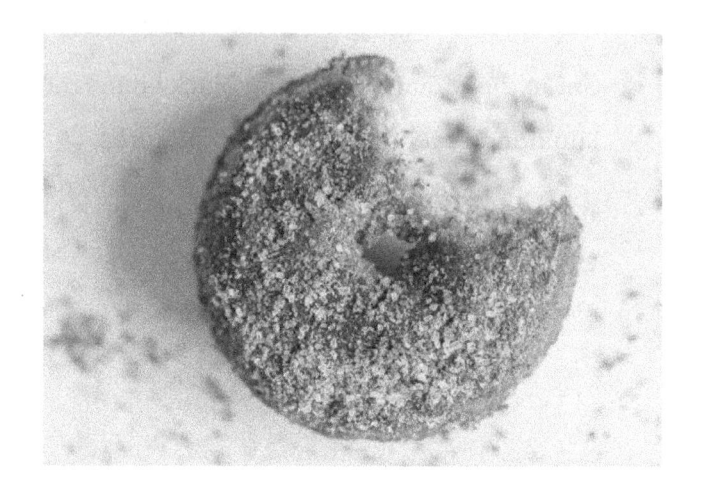

Prep time: 5 mins
Cook time: 25 mins
Carbs per meal: 11g

Ingredients

Donut recipe

1. 11 1/2 ounces cream cheese (room temperature)

2. 1/2 cup extra virgin olive oil
3. 1/4 cup heavy whipping cream
4. 4 large eggs
5. 1/2 teaspoon liquid stevia extract
6. 1/2 teaspoon maple extract
7. 1/2 teaspoon vanilla extract 1/4 cup coconut flour
8. 2 tablespoons coconut flour
9. 2 teaspoons ground cinnamon
10. 1 teaspoon baking powder
11. 1 teaspoon xanthan gum
12. 1/2 teaspoon pink Himalayan salt
13. Topping recipe
14. 1/4 cup So Nourished granular erythritol
15. 1/4 cup ground cinnamon

Instructions

- Preheat the oven to 400 degrees Fahrenheit and grease a 6-cavity donut pan with coconut oil spray.

- In a large bowl, beat the cream cheese, olive oil, cream eggs, stevia and extract using a hand mixer until smooth and fully incorporated. Set aside.

- In a small bowl, whisk together the coconut flour, cinnamon, baking powder, xanthan gum, and salt using a whisk, Add the dry mixture to the wet ingredients and combine using the hand mixer. Fill the greased cavities of the donut mold to the brim, making sure not to overfill.

- Bake for 15 minutes, until the donuts are puffed up and a toothpick comes out clean.

- Meanwhile, put the ingredients for the topping on a plate and combine using your fingers. After removing the donuts from the oven, allow to cool in the pan for 5 minutes then toss them, one at a time, in the cinnamonsugar mixture. Set the coated donuts on a wire baking rack to cool for an additional 6 minutes prior to eating.

COOKIE DOUGH RECIPE NO EGGS

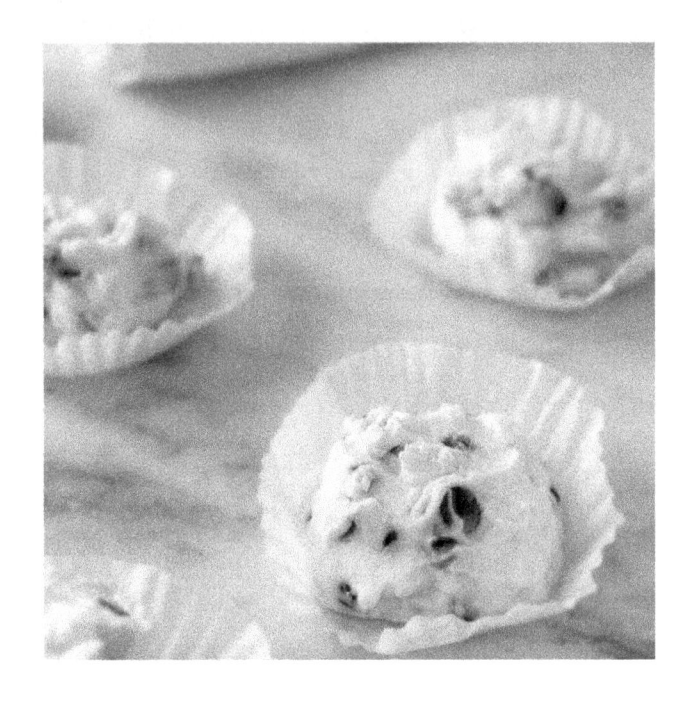

Prep time: 10 mins
Carbs per meal: 19g

Ingredients

1. 1 (8-ounce) package cream cheese (softened)

2. 6 1/2 tablespoons butter (softened)
3. 3 tablespoons So Nourished powdered erythritol
4. 1 teaspoon vanilla extract
5. 1/2 cup Lily's Chocolate Chips

Instructions

- Beat together the cream cheese, butter, powdered erythritol, and vanilla in a bowl.
- Mix on medium speed until light and fluffy.
- Fold in the chocolate chips then spoon into an airtight container and refrigerate to store.

ALMOND MILK ICE CREAM RECIPE

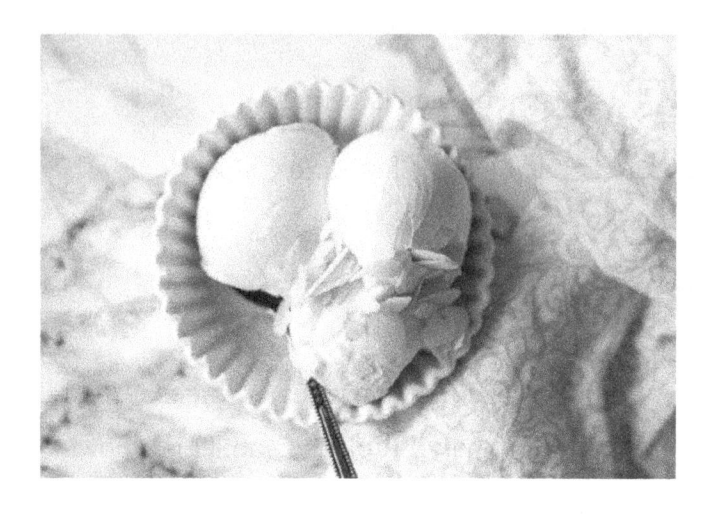

Prep time: 10 mins
Carbs per meal: 33g

Ingredients

1. 4 cups unsweetened almond milk
2. 1/2 cup So Nourished powdered erythritol 1 tablespoon vanilla extract Pinch salt liquid stevia (to taste)

Instructions

- Whisk together the almond milk and erythritol in a medium saucepan over medium heat.

- Stir frequently until the almond milk is steaming then remove from heat.

- Whisk in the vanilla extract and salt along with the liquid stevia extract to taste then cool to room temperature.

- Pour the mixture into a container and freeze until solid.

- Defrost the ice cream for 10 minutes before scooping to serve.

CHEWY GRANOLA BAR RECIPE

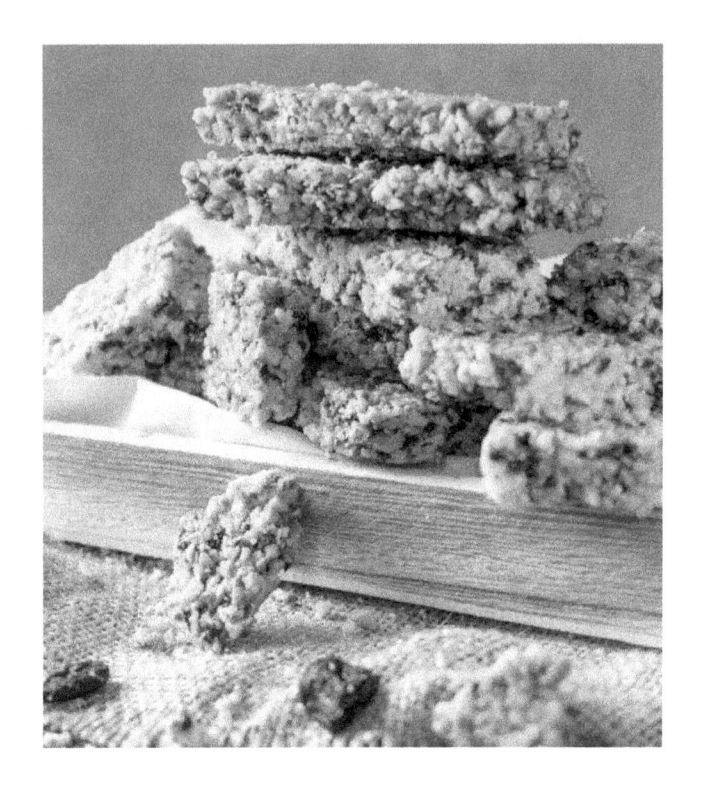

Prep time: 5 minutes
Cook time: 25 minutes
Carbs per meal: 12g

Ingredients

1. 1 1/2 cups sliced almonds

2. 1/2 cup flaked coconut (unsweetened)

3. 1/2 cup pecans

4. 1/2 cup sunflower seeds

5. 1/2 cup dried, unsweetened cranberries (chopped)

6. 1/2 cup butter

7. 1/2 cup So Nourished powdered erythritol

8. 1/2 tsp vanilla extract

9. 1 pinch salt

Instructions

- Preheat the oven to 300°F and line a square baking dish with parchment.

- Combine the almonds, coconut, pecans, and sunflower seeds in a food processor.

- Pulse the mixture until finely chopped and crumb-like, like granola.

- Pour the mixture into a bowl and stir in the cranberries and a pinch of salt.

- Melt the butter in a saucepan over low heat then whisk in the erythritol and vanilla extract.

- Pour the mixture over the granola and stir until well combined.

- Press the mixture into the prepared dish, compacting it as much as possible, and bake for 25 minutes.

- Cool the mixture in the pan completely then remove and cut into 16 bars.

BLUEBERRY COCONUT PORRIDGE

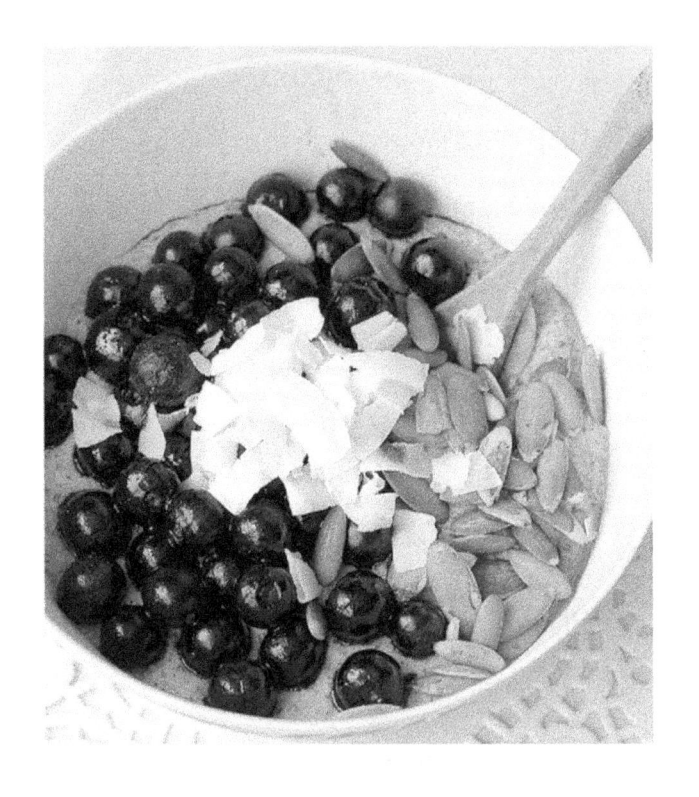

Prep Time: 5 mins
Cook Time: 5 mins
Carbs per meal: 16g

Ingredients

Porridge

1. 1 cup almond milk
2. 1/4 cup ground flaxseed
3. 1/4 cup coconut flour
4. 1 tsp cinnamon
5. 1 tsp vanilla extract
6. 10 drops liquid stevia
7. pinch salt

Toppings

8. tbsp butter
9. 60 grams blueberries
10. 2 tbsp pumpkin seeds
11. 1 oz. shaved coconut

Instructions

- Set a cup of almond milk to heat up on a low flame.

- Add in flaxseed, coconut flour, cinnamon and salt. Use a whisk to break up any clumps.

- Heat until slightly bubbling. Add in liquid stevia and vanilla extract.

- When the mixture is as thick as you want it to be, turn off the flame and add in your toppings. We like to add cold butter, fresh or frozen blueberries, pumpkin seeds and shaved coconut!

BLINI STYLE CAVIAR CREPES

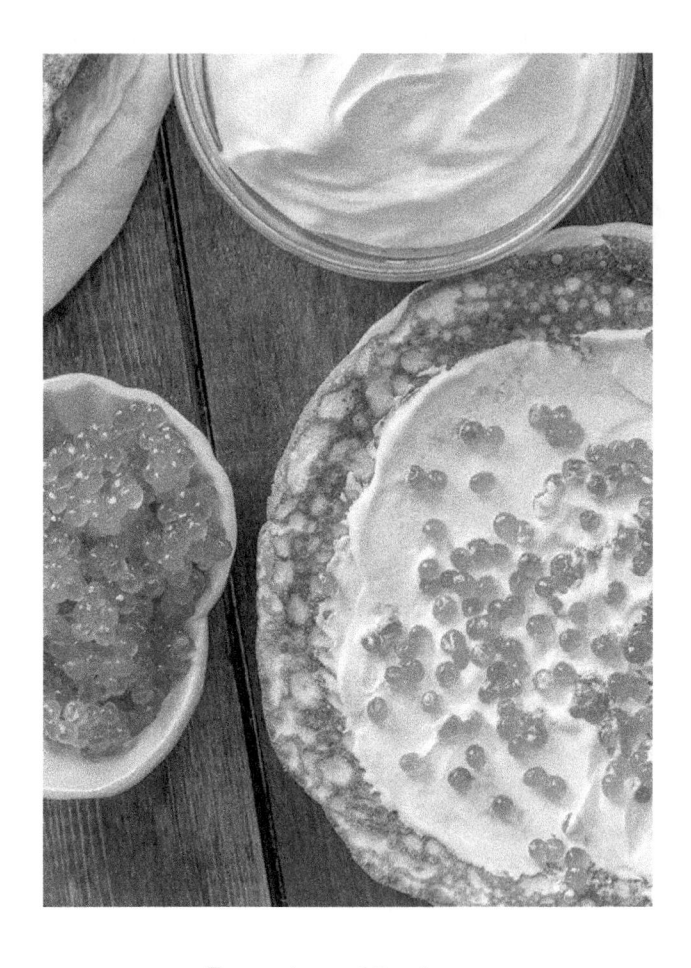

Prep time: 10 minutes
Cook time: 10 minutes
Carbs per meal: 15g

Ingredients

Blini

1. 2 oz. cream cheese
2. 2 large eggs
3. 1/2 tsp baking powder
4. 1 pinch sea salt

Filling

5. 1/2 cup sour cream
6. 3/4 cup wild Alaskan salmon caviar

Instructions

- Prepare the blini style crepes by combining all the ingredients in a food processor or blender and blending until smooth.

- Heat up a small skillet with a bit of butter on medium heat. Let it heat up fully! Ladle a little less than 1/4 cup of batter in at a time and swirl the contents around to spread it evenly. Cook until the edges start to peel away from the skillet and bubbles have formed on top. This should take about 2-3 minutes per crepe. Flip and cook for another minute. Repeat with all the batter. This recipe should make 4 medium sized crepes.

- Once the batter has cooked and the crepes are ready, spoon 2 tablespoons of sour cream onto each, followed by 2-3 tablespoons of wild Alaskan salmon caviar. Roll each up and enjoy!

PUMPKIN MACADAMIA BUTTER

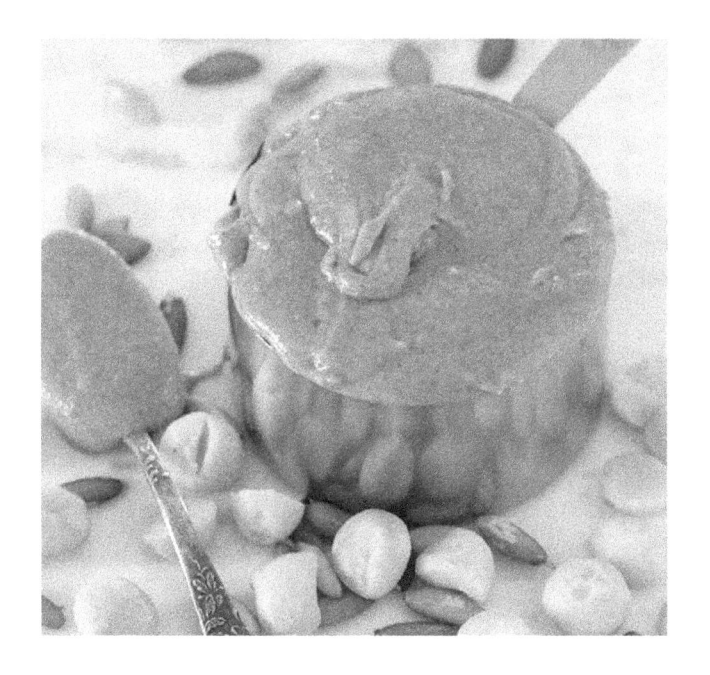

Prep Time: 10 mins
Carbs per meal: 6g

Ingredients

1. 2 cups pumpkin seeds

2. 1 cup macadamia nuts

3. 10 drops liquid stevia

4. 1/4 tsp sea salt

Instructions

- Combine all the ingredients in a food processor and blend until smooth and creamy.
- Taste and adjust the sweetness and saltiness, if desired.
- Store in an airtight container in the refrigerator for 2-4 weeks.

BRIE & APPLE CREPES

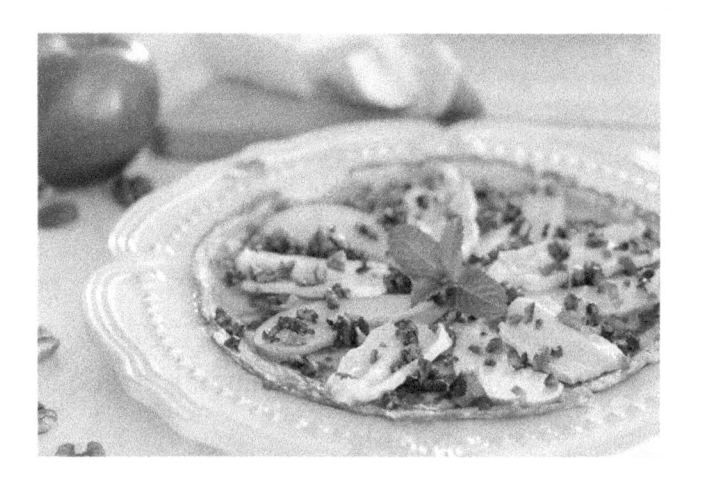

Prep time: 5 mins
Cook time: 15 mins
Carbs per meal: 23g

Ingredients

Crepe Batter

1. 4 oz. cream cheese
2. 4 large eggs
3. 1/2 tsp baking soda

4. 1/4 tsp sea salt

Toppings

5. 2 oz. chopped pecans
6. 1 tbsp unsalted butter
7. 1/4 tsp cinnamon
8. 1 small gala apple (or any sweet apple) 4 oz. brie cheese (room temperature) fresh mint leaves (for garnish)

<u>Instructions</u>

- Begin by combining the batter ingredients in a Nutribullet or blender and blending until smooth.

- Heat up a small amount of unsalted butter in a non-stick pan on medium heat. Ladle some of the crepe batter into the pan and swirl the contents around so that the batter is thin and spread out evenly. Let cook until the top looks dry (about 23 minutes), then flip gently with a large spatula and cook the other side for a few seconds.

- Repeat this step until you have about 12 crepes. Layer them on top of each other on a plate while you prep the toppings/fillings.

- Melt a tablespoon of butter in a small pan and toast the chopped pecans until fragrant, but not too browned. Sprinkle with cinnamon and mix. Then, transfer them to a plate to cool.

- Slice an apple thinly, as well as the brie cheese.

- Arrange the apple slices and brie on 1 crepe and top with some of the toasted pecans. Repeat for all the crepes until all the toppings have been used.

- Garnish with mint and enjoy with a fork and knife or rolled up!

Grandma's Honey Muffins

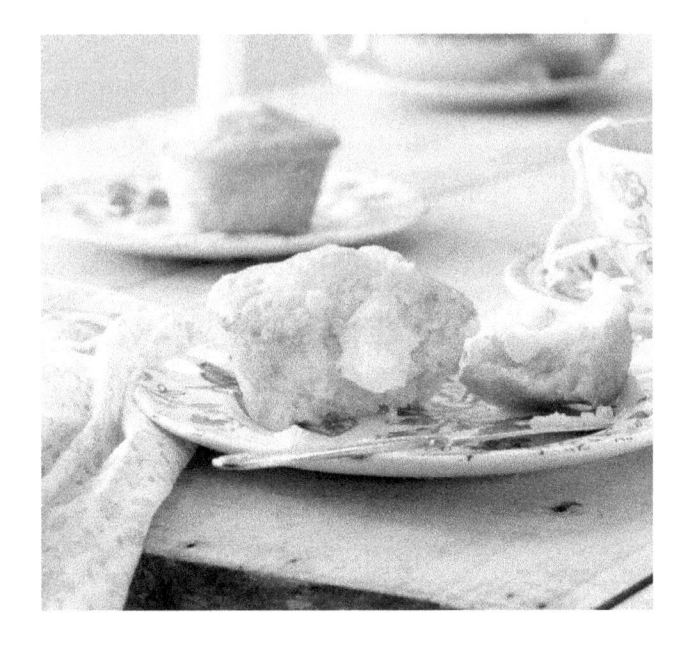

*Prep/Total Time: 30 min.
Carbs per meal: 31g*

Ingredients

1. 2 cups all-purpose flour

2. 1/2 cup sugar

3. 3 teaspoons baking powder

4. 1/2 teaspoon salt

5. 1 large Eggland's Best egg, room temperature

6. 1 cup 2% milk

7. 1/4 cup butter, melted

8. 1/4 cup honey

INSTRUCTIONS:

- Preheat oven to 400°. In a large bowl, combine flour, sugar, baking powder and salt. In a small bowl, combine egg, milk, butter and honey. Stir into dry ingredients just until moistened.

- Fill greased or paper-lined muffin cups three-fourths full. Bake until a toothpick inserted in center comes out clean, 15-18 minutes. Cool 5 minutes before removing from pan to a wire rack. Serve warm.

- Freeze option: Freeze cooled muffins in freezer containers. To use, thaw at room temperature or, if desired, microwave each muffin on high until heated through, 20-30 seconds.

Taco Cracker

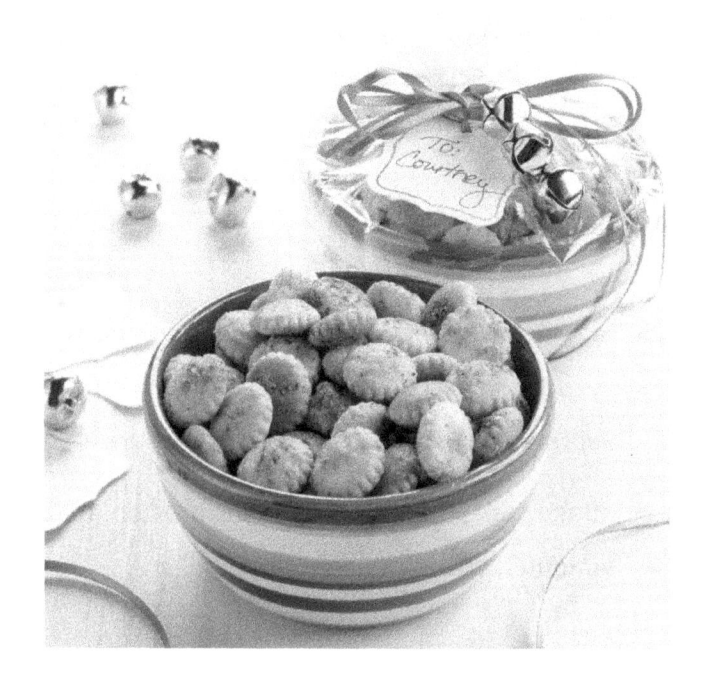

Prep/Total Time: 30 min.
Carbs per meal: 21g

Ingredients

1. 3 packages (10 ounces each) oyster crackers
2. 3/4 cup canola oil

3. 1 envelope taco seasoning

4. 1/2 teaspoon garlic powder

5. 1/2 teaspoon dried oregano

6. 1/2 teaspoon chili powder

INSTRUCTIONS:

- Place the crackers in a large roasting pan; drizzle with oil. Combine the seasonings; sprinkle over crackers and toss to coat.

- Bake at 350° until golden brown, 15-20 minutes, stirring once.

LEMON AND THYME CHICKEN THIGHS

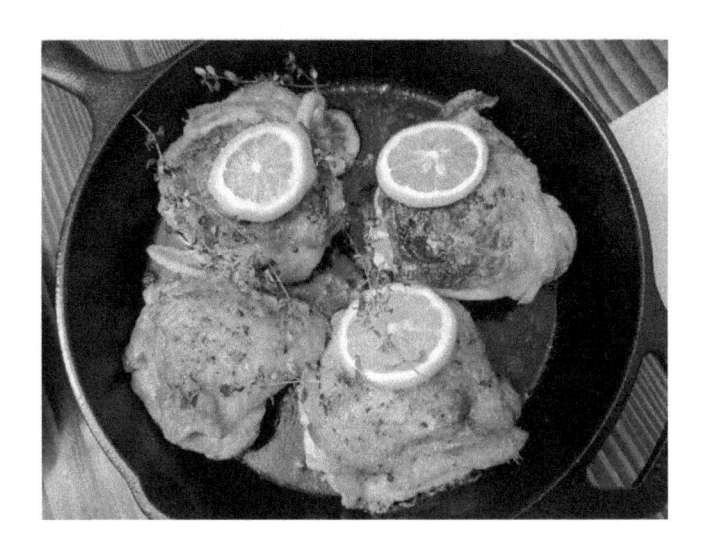

This recipe highlights how great high-quality chicken can taste when combined with just a little seasoning, fresh herbs and lemon juice. This combination allows the chicken to stay very moist, tender and full of nutrients. Ideal as a meal, snack or even as a picnic dish the following day.

Prep time: 5 mins

Cook time: 30 mins
Carbs per meal: 18g

Ingredients

1. 6 bone-in, skin-on chicken thighs (2 pounds)
2. ½ teaspoon fine sea salt
3. ½ teaspoon ground black pepper
4. ½ teaspoon garlic powder
5. 1 tablespoon ghee, lard or tallow
6. 1 large lemon, sliced
7. 6 sprigs of fresh thyme
8. 1 tablespoon freshly squeezed lemon juice

INSTRUCTIONS

- Preheat the oven to 450°F.
- Sprinkle the chicken on both sides with the salt, pepper, and garlic powder then heat the ghee in a large cast-iron skillet over medium-

high heat then place the chicken thighs in the pan, skin side down, and cook for 2 minutes.

- Reduce the heat to medium and continue cooking the thighs without touching them for another 10 minutes, or until the skin has released from the pan (the skin will initially stick to the pan and then will release once the fat has rendered).

- Drain any excess fat from the pan, then transfer the skillet to the oven (remember, the handle will be hot).

- Cook for 10 more minutes.

- Remove the skillet from the oven and flip the chicken pieces over and then nestle the lemon slices and thyme sprigs between the chicken pieces, then return the pan to the oven for 5 minutes, or until the skin is crispy and the juices run clear when a knife is inserted and the meat is no longer pink inside, or the internal temperature of the chicken reaches 165°F.

- Remove from the oven. Drizzle with lemon juice, and serve.

PLANT BASED RECIPES

Vegetarian Tortilla Soup

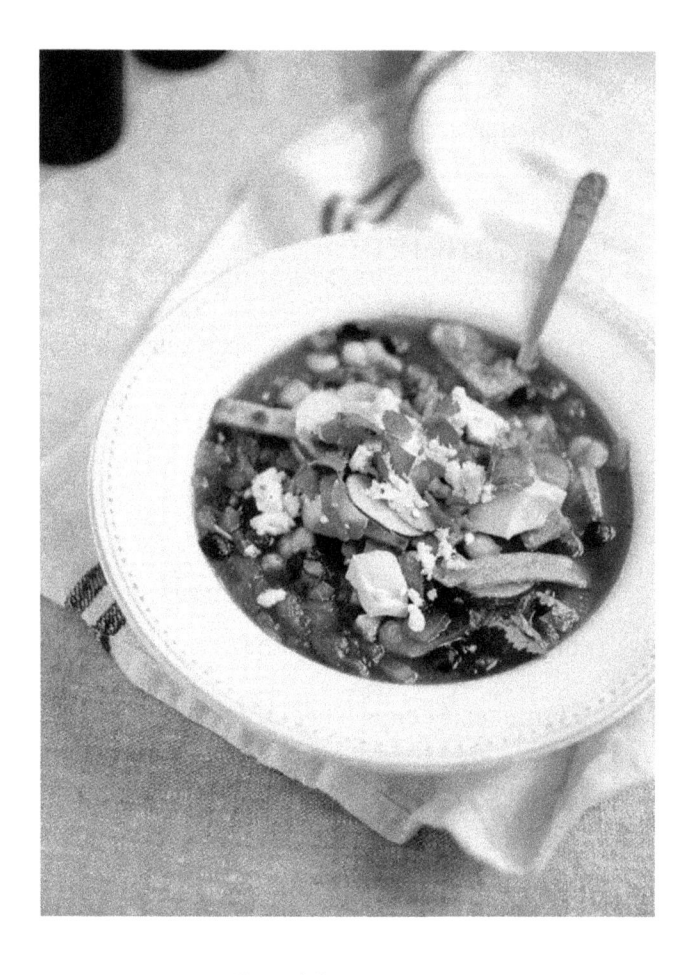

- *Prep Time: 10 mins*

- *Cook Time: 20 mins*

INGREDIENTS:

1. 1 dried smoked chili pepper or 1 poblano pepper
2. Olive oil
3. 1 medium white onion, diced
4. 2 cloves garlic, pressed or minced.
5. 1 to 2 medium jalapeños (optional, use one for medium spicy soup and two for spicy soup)
6. 1 teaspoon ground cumin
7. 14-ounce can crushed tomatoes or chunky tomato sauce*
8. 32 ounces (4 cups) vegetable stock
9. 14-ounce can hominy, rinsed and drained (optional)
10. 14-ounce can black beans, rinsed and drained
11. Sea salt

12. 6 corn tortillas (6-inch, taco-sized)

13. 1 avocado

14. 2 to 4 radishes, sliced into super thin rounds

15. 2 ounces queso fresco or feta cheese (optional), crumbled

16. 1 handful cilantro leaves, chopped

17. 1 lime, sliced into small wedges

INSTRUCTIONS:

- Prep work: Preheat the oven to 475 degrees Fahrenheit. Stack the tortillas and slice them into ½-inch-wide, 2-inch-long strips. Remove the seeds and membranes from the jalapeno (and poblano, if using) and chop the peppers. Wash your hands. Pit, peel, and medium dice the avocado, then squeeze some lime juice over the avocado to prevent browning.

- Bake the tortillas: Coat a baking sheet with a thin layer of oil. Toss the tortilla strips in the oil to coat and arrange the strips in a single layer. Bake 6 to 8 minutes, or until golden brown. While the strips are hot, season them with salt.

- Toast the chili pepper: Place the dried chili pepper onto a baking sheet and bake for about 1 minute, or until the pepper is warmed through. When cool enough to handle, cut the pepper open and remove the seeds. (Wash your hands afterward and avoid touching your eyes!)

- Make the soup: In a medium pot or Dutch oven, heat some olive oil on medium until hot. Add the onion, garlic, jalapeno and poblano peppers (if using). Cook 4 to 5 minutes, or until softened, stirring occasionally. Stir in the cumin, then the canned tomatoes and vegetable stock. Simmer for about 3 minutes, then add the hominy, black beans and the seeded chili pepper. Cook for 8 to 10 minutes, or until slightly thickened, stirring occasionally. Season with salt and pepper to taste.

- Serve the soup: First, discard the dried chili pepper. Place some of the avocado, radishes, tortilla strips, and queso fresco (or feta) at the bottom of 2 to 4 bowls. Divide the soup between the bowls. Top the soup with the remaining avocado, radishes, tortilla strips, and queso fresco (or feta). Garnish with some cilantro and serve with lime wedges and hot sauce, if desired.

Sweet Potato and Black Bean Tacos

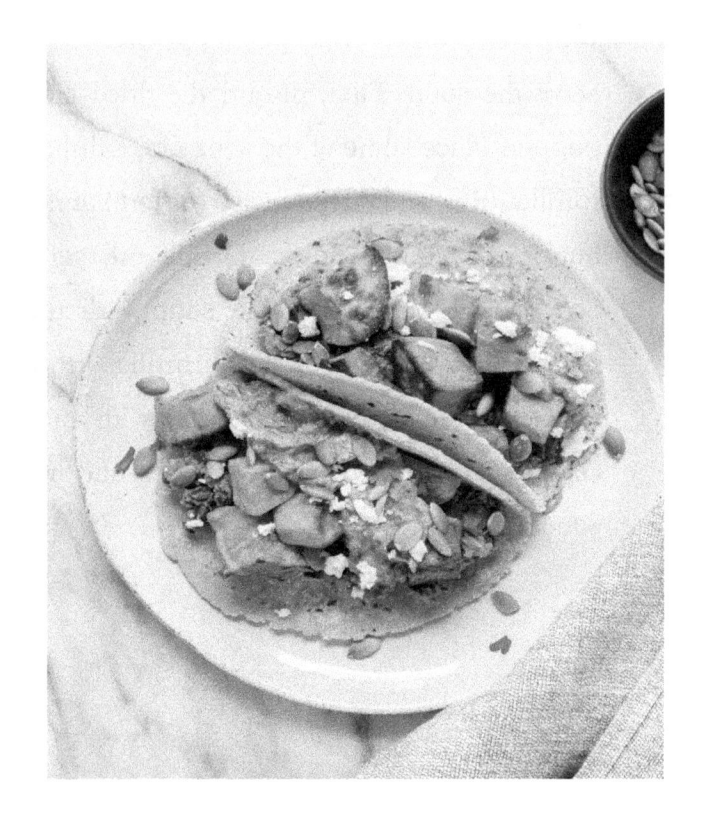

Prep Time: 30 mins
Cook Time: 30 mins

INGREDIENTS:

Sweet potatoes

1. 2 pounds sweet potatoes (3 to 4 medium sweet potatoes), peeled and sliced into 1-inch chunks
2. 2 tablespoons olive oil
3. ¼ teaspoon cayenne pepper (omit if sensitive to spice)
4. ¼ teaspoon fine sea salt

Spicy black beans

1. 1 tablespoon olive oil
2. 1 small yellow or white onion, finely chopped
3. Fine sea salt
4. 2 teaspoons ground cumin
5. ¼ teaspoon chili powder
6. 2 cans black beans, rinsed and drained (or 3 cups cooked black beans)
7. ⅓ cup water
8. 1 teaspoon sherry vinegar or lime juice

9. Freshly ground black pepper, to taste

Avocado-pepita dip

1. 2 avocados, pitted
2. 1 cup lightly packed fresh cilantro (mostly leaves, some small stems are ok)
3. ½ cup pepitas
4. 1 small jalapeño, seeded and roughly chopped, or ¼ teaspoon red pepper flakes (go easy if sensitive to spice)
5. 2 cloves garlic, roughly chopped
6. 2 tablespoons lime juice (about 1 medium lime) or 1 tablespoon sherry vinegar
7. 2 tablespoons water
8. ½ teaspoon fine grain sea salt
9. Freshly ground black pepper, to taste

Everything else

1. 8 to 10 small corn tortillas

2. Crumbled feta

3. Suggested garnishes: Pickled jalapeños or pickled radishes or pickled red onions, torn cilantro, hot sauce, etc.

INSTRUCTIONS:

- Roast the sweet potatoes: Preheat the oven to 425 degrees Fahrenheit and line a large, rimmed baking sheet with parchment paper for easy clean-up. Toss the prepared sweet potatoes with the olive oil, cayenne pepper (if using) and salt. Arrange in a single layer and bake for 30 to 40 minutes, tossing halfway, until the sweet potatoes are tender and caramelizing at the edges.

- Prepare the black beans: Warm the olive oil in a large saucepan over medium heat. Add the onions and a sprinkle of salt. Cook, stirring occasionally, until the onions have softened and are turning translucent, about 5 to 8 minutes. Add the cumin and chili powder and cook for about 30 seconds while stirring. Pour in the beans and water. Stir, cover and reduce heat to maintain a gentle simmer.

- Cook for 5 minutes, then remove the lid and use a potato masher or a fork to mash up at least half of the beans. Remove from heat, stir in the vinegar, season with salt (I added over ¼ teaspoon) and pepper, and cover until you're ready to serve.

- Make the avocado dip: First, toast the pepitas in a skillet over medium heat, stirring often, until they are fragrant and starting to make little popping noises, about 5 minutes. Transfer to a bowl and set aside.

- Scoop the avocado flesh into a food processor or blender. Add the cilantro, jalapeño, garlic, lime juice, water and salt. Blend until smooth, scraping down the sides of the processor/blender as necessary. Add almost all of the pepitas (reserve a few tablespoons for garnish) and process just until the pepitas are chopped into small pieces (some remaining texture is desirable). Taste, and add more salt if necessary. Transfer the dip to a small bowl for serving.

- To warm the tortillas, heat a large skillet over medium heat and warm the tortillas in batches, flipping to warm each side. Alternatively, you can warm them directly over a low flame on a gas range. Stack the warmed tortillas on a plate and cover with a tea towel to keep warm.

- To assemble the tacos, spread black beans down the middle of each tortilla, then top with some sweet potatoes and avocado-pepita dip. Garnish with feta, pepitas, and anything else that strikes your fancy. Repeat with remaining tortillas and serve.

Grilled Cauliflower Wedges

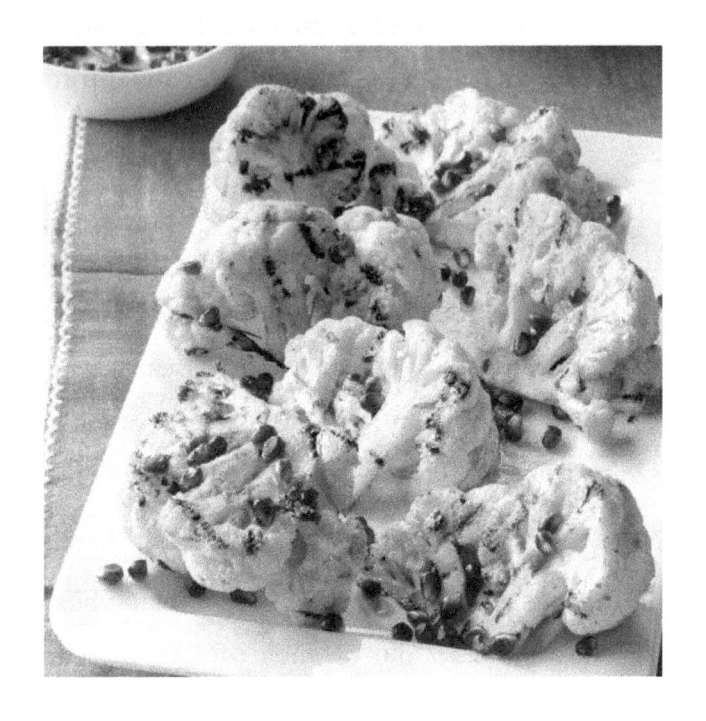

Total Time
Prep/Total Time: 30 min.

INGREDIENTS:

1. 1 large head cauliflower
2. 1 teaspoon ground turmeric

3. 1/2 teaspoon crushed red pepper flakes
4. 2 tablespoons olive oil
5. Lemon juice, additional olive oil and pomegranate seeds, optional

INSTRUCTIONS:

- Remove leaves and trim stem from cauliflower. Cut cauliflower into eight wedges. Mix turmeric and pepper flakes. Brush wedges with oil; sprinkle with turmeric mixture.

- Grill, covered, over medium-high heat or broil 4 in. from heat until cauliflower is tender, 8-10 minutes on each side. If desired, drizzle with lemon juice and additional oil and serve with pomegranate seeds.

Roasted Balsamic Red Potatoes

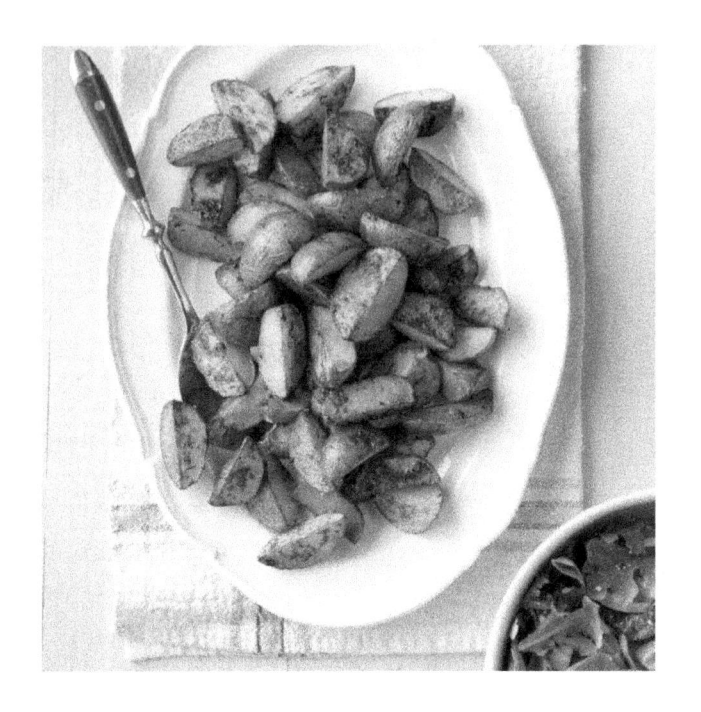

Total Time
Prep: 10 min. Bake: 30 min.

Ingredients:

1. 2 pounds small red potatoes, cut into wedges

2. 2 tablespoons olive oil

3. 3/4 teaspoon garlic pepper blend

4. 1/2 teaspoon Italian seasoning

5. 1/4 teaspoon salt

6. 1/4 cup balsamic vinegar

7. Preheat oven to 425°. Toss potatoes with oil and seasonings; spread in a 15x10x1-in. pan.

8. Roast 25 minutes, stirring halfway. Drizzle with vinegar; roast until potatoes are tender, 5-10 minutes.

Easy Homemade Chunky Applesauce

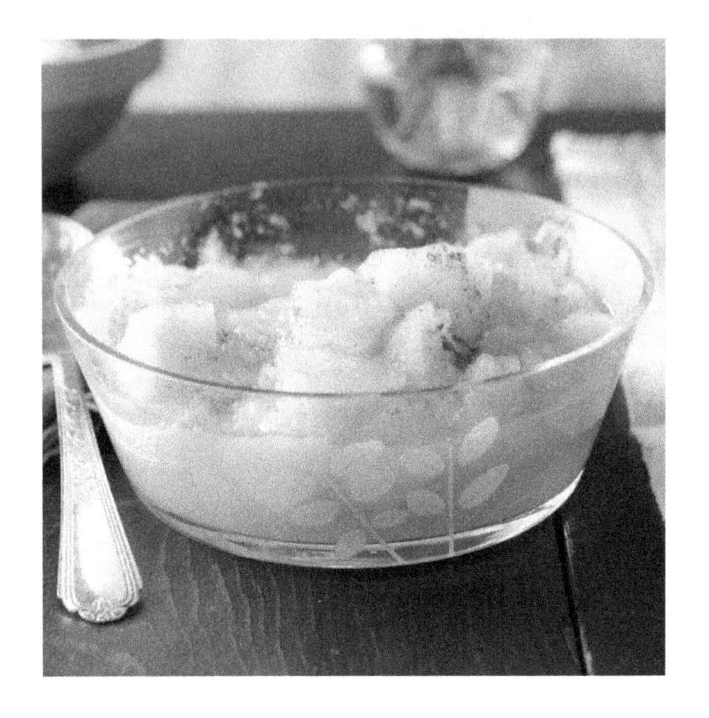

Total Time
Prep/Total Time: 30 min.

Ingredients:

1. 7 medium McIntosh, Empire or other apples (about 3 pounds)
2. 1/2 cup sugar

3. 1/2 cup water

4. 1 tablespoon lemon juice

5. 1/4 teaspoon almond or vanilla extract

INSTRUCTIONS:

- Peel, core and cut each apple into 8 wedges. Cut each wedge crosswise in half; place in a large saucepan. Add remaining ingredients.
- Bring to a boil. Reduce heat; simmer, covered, until desired consistency is reached, 15-20 minutes, stirring occasionally.

Black Bean-Tomato Chi

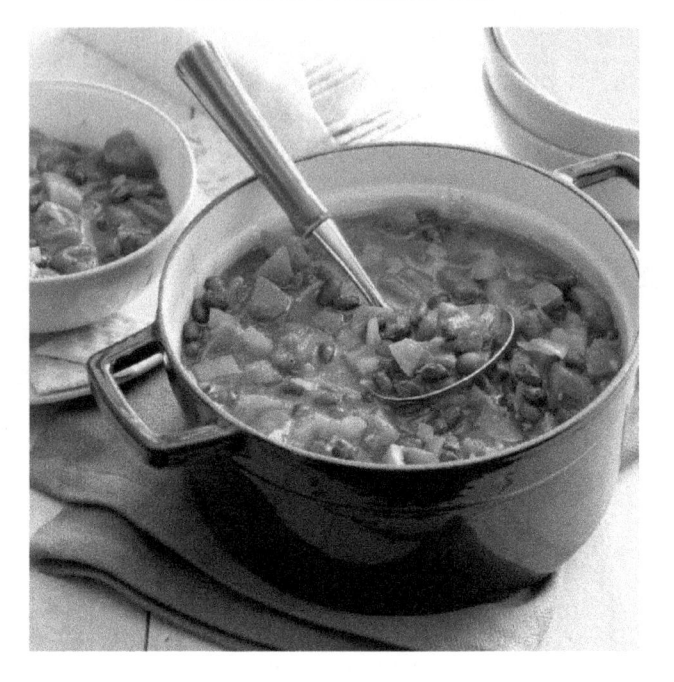

Total Time
Prep: 10 min. Cook: 35 min.

Ingredients:

1. 2 tablespoons olive oil
2. 1 large onion, chopped
3. 1 medium green pepper, chopped

4. 3 garlic cloves, minced
5. 1 teaspoon ground cinnamon
6. 1 teaspoon ground cumin
7. 1 teaspoon chili powder
8. 1/4 teaspoon pepper
9. 3 cans (14-1/2 ounces each) diced tomatoes, undrained
10. 2 cans (15 ounces each) black beans, rinsed and drained
11. 1 cup orange juice or juice from 3 medium oranges

INSTRUCTIONS:

- In a Dutch oven, heat oil over medium-high heat. Add onion and green pepper; cook and stir 8-10 minutes or until tender. Add garlic and seasonings; cook 1 minute longer.

- Stir in remaining ingredients; bring to a boil. Reduce heat; simmer, covered, 20-25 minutes to allow flavors to blend, stirring occasionally.

Mushroom & Broccoli Soup

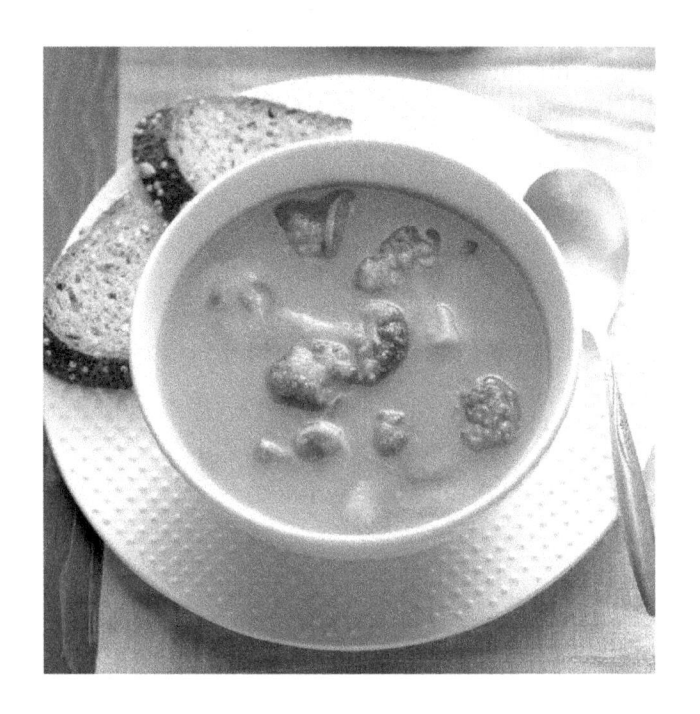

Total Time
Prep: 20 min. Cook: 45 min.

Ingredients:

1. 1 bunch broccoli (about 1-1/2 pounds)
2. 1 tablespoon canola oil

3. 1/2 pound sliced fresh mushrooms

4. 1 tablespoon reduced-sodium soy sauce

5. 2 medium carrots, finely chopped

6. 2 celery ribs, finely chopped

7. 1/4 cup finely chopped onion

8. 1 garlic clove, minced

9. 1 carton (32 ounces) vegetable broth

10. 2 cups water

11. 2 tablespoons lemon juice

INSTRUCTIONS:

- Cut broccoli florets into bite-size pieces. Peel and chop stalks.

- In a large saucepan, heat oil over medium-high heat; saute mushrooms until tender, 4-6 minutes. Stir in soy sauce; remove from pan.

- In same pan, combine broccoli stalks, carrots, celery, onion, garlic, broth and water; bring to a boil. Reduce heat; simmer, uncovered, until vegetables are softened, 25-30 minutes.

- Puree soup using an immersion blender. Or, cool slightly and puree soup in a blender; return to pan. Stir in florets and mushrooms; bring to a boil. Reduce heat to medium; cook until broccoli is tender, 8-10 minutes, stirring occasionally. Stir in lemon juice.

Avocado Fruit Salad with Tangerine Vinaigrette

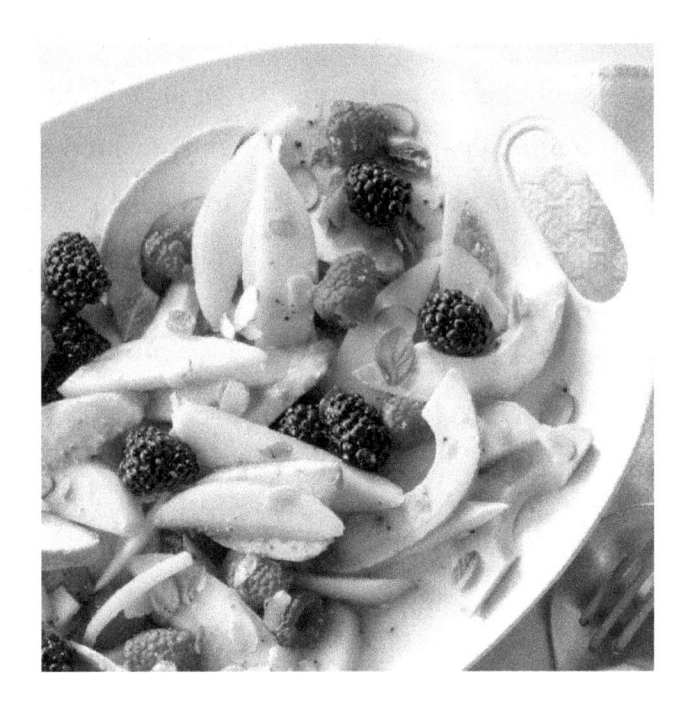

Total Time
Prep/Total Time: 25 min.

Ingredients:

1. 3 medium ripe avocados, peeled and thinly sliced

2. 3 medium mangoes, peeled and thinly sliced
3. 1 cup fresh raspberries
4. 1 cup fresh blackberries
5. 1/4 cup minced fresh mint
6. 1/4 cup sliced almonds, toasted
7. DRESSING:
8. 1/2 cup olive oil
9. 1 teaspoon grated tangerine or orange peel
10. 1/4 cup tangerine or orange juice
11. 2 tablespoons balsamic vinegar
12. 1/2 teaspoon salt
13. 1/4 teaspoon freshly ground pepper

INSTRUCTIONS:

- Arrange avocados and fruit on a serving plate; sprinkle with mint and almonds. In a small bowl, whisk dressing ingredients until blended; drizzle over salad

- Note: To toast nuts, bake in a shallow pan in a 350° oven for 5-10 minutes or cook in a skillet over low heat until lightly browned, stirring occasionally.

Roasted Curried Chickpeas and Cauliflower

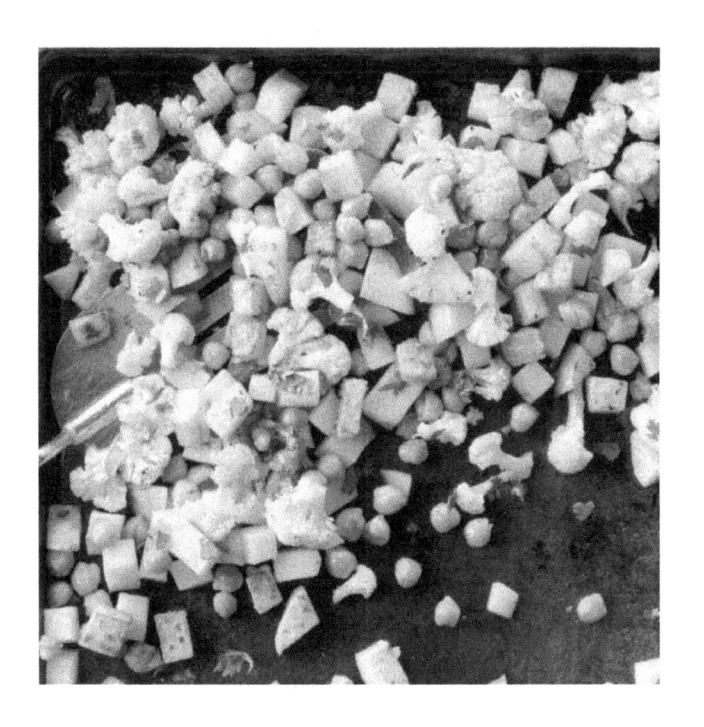

Total Time
Prep: 15 min. Bake: 30 min.

Ingredients:

1. 2 pounds potatoes (about 4 medium), peeled and cut into 1/2-inch cubes

2. 1 small head cauliflower, broken into florets (about 3 cups)
3. 1 can (15 ounces) chickpeas, rinsed and drained
4. 3 tablespoons olive oil
5. 2 teaspoons curry powder
6. 3/4 teaspoon salt
7. 1/4 teaspoon pepper
8. 3 tablespoons minced fresh cilantro or parsley

INSTRUCTIONS:

- Preheat oven to 400°. Place first 7 ingredients in a large bowl; toss to coat. Transfer to a 15x10x1-in. baking pan coated with cooking spray.
- Roast until vegetables are tender, 30-35 minutes, stirring occasionally. Sprinkle with cilantro.

Chickpea Mint Tabbouleh

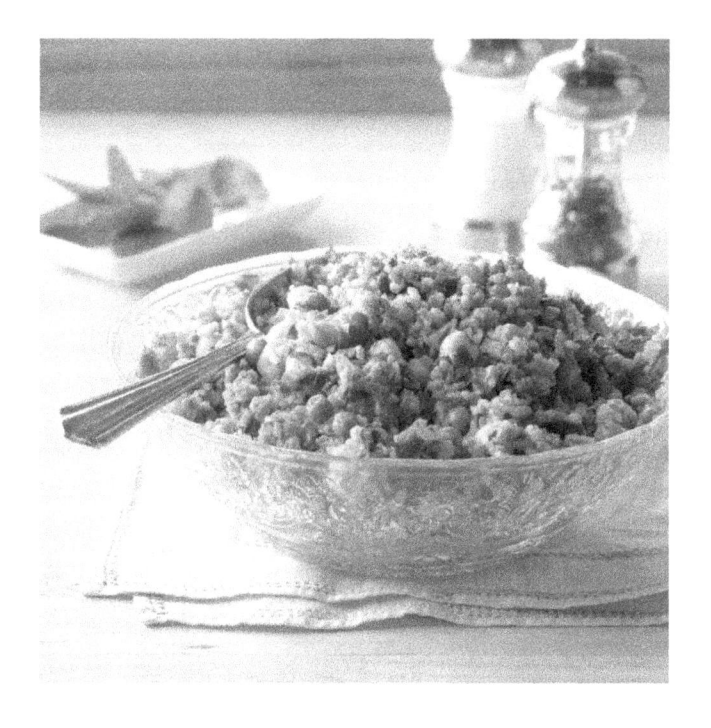

Total Time
Prep/Total Time: 30 min

Ingredients:

1. 1 cup bulgur
2. 2 cups water

3. 1 cup fresh or frozen peas (about 5 ounces), thawed

4. 1 can (15 ounces) chickpeas or garbanzo beans, rinsed and drained

5. 1/2 cup minced fresh parsley

6. 1/4 cup minced fresh mint

7. 1/4 cup olive oil

8. 2 tablespoons julienned soft sun-dried tomatoes (not packed in oil)

9. 2 tablespoons lemon juice

10. 1/2 teaspoon salt

11. 1/4 teaspoon pepper

INSTRUCTIONS:

- In a large saucepan, combine bulgur and water; bring to a boil. Reduce heat; simmer, covered, 10 minutes. Stir in fresh or frozen peas; cook, covered, until bulgur and peas are tender, about 5 minutes.

- Transfer to a large bowl. Stir in remaining ingredients. Serve warm or refrigerate and serve cold.

- Editor's Note: This recipe was tested with soft sun-dried tomatoes that do not need to be soaked before use.

- Health Tip: Bulgur is made from whole wheat kernels that are boiled, dried and cracked. Since it's made from the whole kernel, it's always a whole grain. It has more fiber than quinoa, oats and corn.

Creamy Cauliflower Pakora Soup

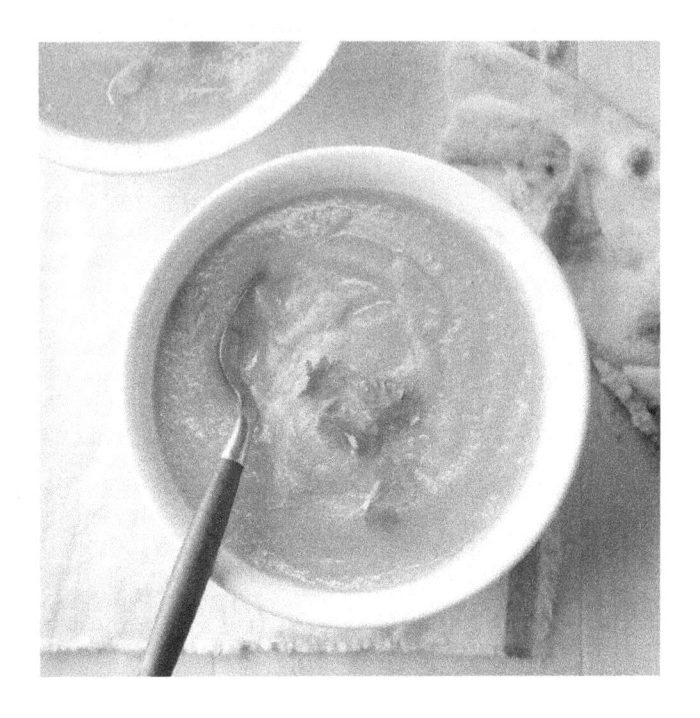

Total Time
Prep: 20 min. Cook: 20 min.

Ingredients:

1. 1 large head cauliflower, cut into small florets
2. 5 medium potatoes, peeled and diced

3. 1 large onion, diced
4. 4 medium carrots, peeled and diced
5. 2 celery ribs, diced
6. 1 carton (32 ounces) vegetable stock
7. 1 teaspoon garam masala
8. 1 teaspoon garlic powder
9. 1 teaspoon ground coriander
10. 1 teaspoon ground turmeric
11. 1 teaspoon ground cumin
12. 1 teaspoon pepper
13. 1 teaspoon salt
14. 1/2 teaspoon crushed red pepper flakes
15. Water or additional vegetable stock
16. Fresh cilantro leaves
17. Lime wedges, optional

INSTRUCTIONS:

- In a Dutch oven over medium-high heat, bring first 14 ingredients to a boil. Cook and stir until vegetables are tender, about 20 minutes. Remove from heat; cool slightly. Process in batches in a blender or food processor until smooth. Adjust consistency as desired with water (or additional stock). Sprinkle with fresh cilantro. Serve hot, with lime wedges if desired.

- Freeze option: Before adding cilantro, freeze cooled soup in freezer containers. To use, partially thaw in refrigerator overnight. Heat through in a saucepan, stirring occasionally and adding a little water if necessary. Sprinkle with cilantro. If desired, serve with lime wedges.

Spice Trade Beans & Bulgur

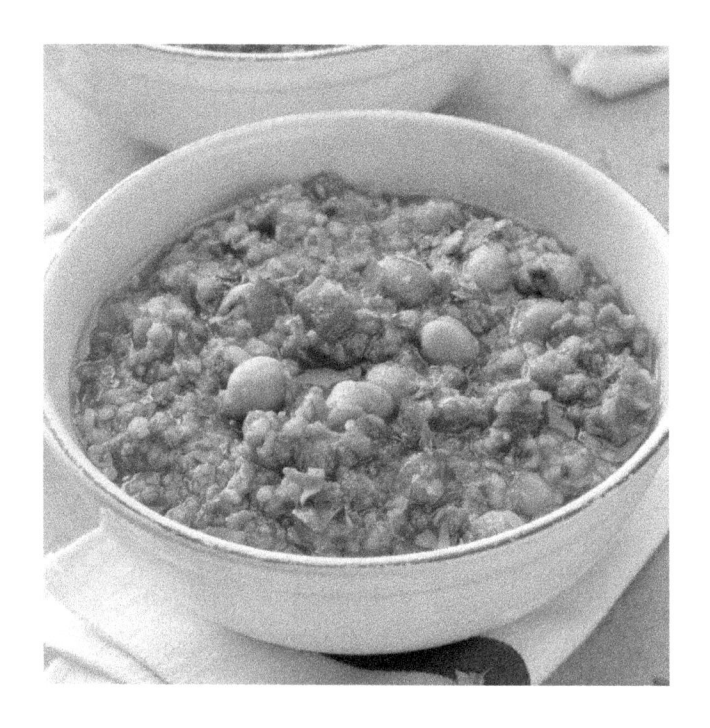

Total Time
Prep: 30 min. Cook: 3-1/2 hours

Ingredients:

1. In a large skillet, heat 2 tablespoons oil over medium-high heat. Add onions and pepper; cook and stir until tender, 3-4 minutes. Add

garlic and seasonings; cook 1 minute longer. Transfer to a 5-qt. slow cooker.

2. In same skillet, heat remaining oil over medium-high heat. Add bulgur; cook and stir until lightly browned, 2-3 minutes or until lightly browned.

3. Add bulgur, tomatoes, broth, brown sugar and soy sauce to slow cooker. Cook, covered, on low 3-4 hours or until bulgur is tender. Stir in beans and raisins; cook 30 minutes longer. If desired, sprinkle with cilantro.

4. 3 tablespoons canola oil, divided

5. 2 medium onions, chopped

6. 1 medium sweet red pepper, chopped

7. 5 garlic cloves, minced

8. 1 tablespoon ground cumin

9. 1 tablespoon paprika

10. 2 teaspoons ground ginger

11. 1 teaspoon pepper

12. 1/2 teaspoon ground cinnamon

13. 1/2 teaspoon cayenne pepper

14. 1-1/2 cups bulgur

15. 1 can (28 ounces) crushed tomatoes

16. 1 can (14-1/2 ounces) diced tomatoes, undrained

17. 1 carton (32 ounces) vegetable broth

18. 2 tablespoons brown sugar

19. 2 tablespoons soy sauce

20. 1 can (15 ounces) garbanzo beans or chickpeas, rinsed and drained

21. **1/2 cup golden raisins**

22. **Minced fresh**

Garden Vegetable & Herb Soup

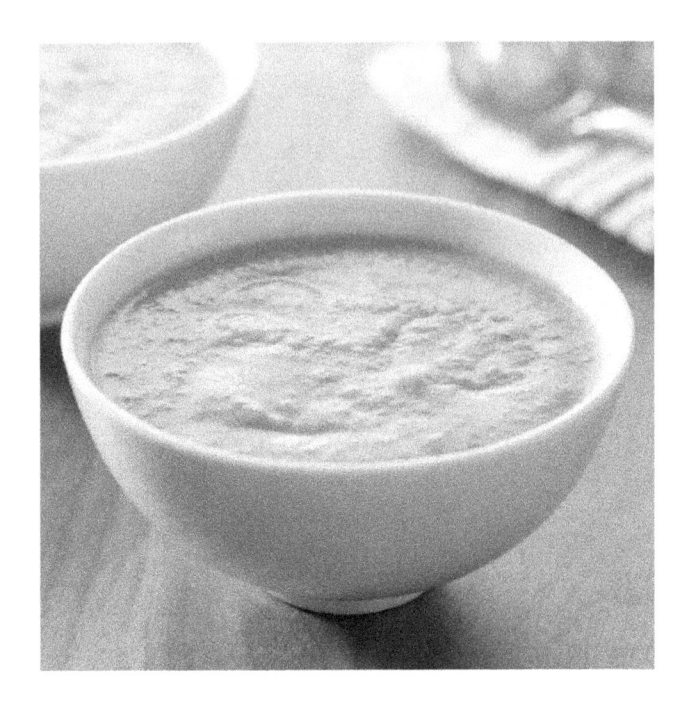

Total Time
Prep: 20 min. Cook: 30 min.

Ingredients:

1. 2 tablespoons olive oil

2. 2 medium onions, chopped

3. 2 large carrots, sliced

4. 1 pound red potatoes (about 3 medium), cubed

5. 2 cups water

6. 1 can (14-1/2 ounces) diced tomatoes in sauce

7. 1-1/2 cups vegetable broth

8. 1-1/2 teaspoons garlic powder

9. 1 teaspoon dried basil

10. 1/2 teaspoon salt

11. 1/2 teaspoon paprika

12. 1/4 teaspoon dill weed

13. 1/4 teaspoon pepper

14. 1 medium yellow summer squash, halved and sliced

15. 1 medium zucchini, halved and sliced

INSTRUCTION:

- In a large saucepan, heat oil over medium heat. Add onions and carrots; cook and stir until onions are tender, 4-6 minutes. Add potatoes and cook 2 minutes. Stir in water, tomatoes, broth and seasonings. Bring to a boil. Reduce heat; simmer, uncovered, until potatoes and carrots are tender, 8-10 minutes.

- Add yellow squash and zucchini; cook until vegetables are tender, 8-10 minutes longer. Serve or, if desired, puree mixture in batches, adding additional broth until desired consistency is achieved.

MEAT BASED RECIPES

Meat Loaf Minia

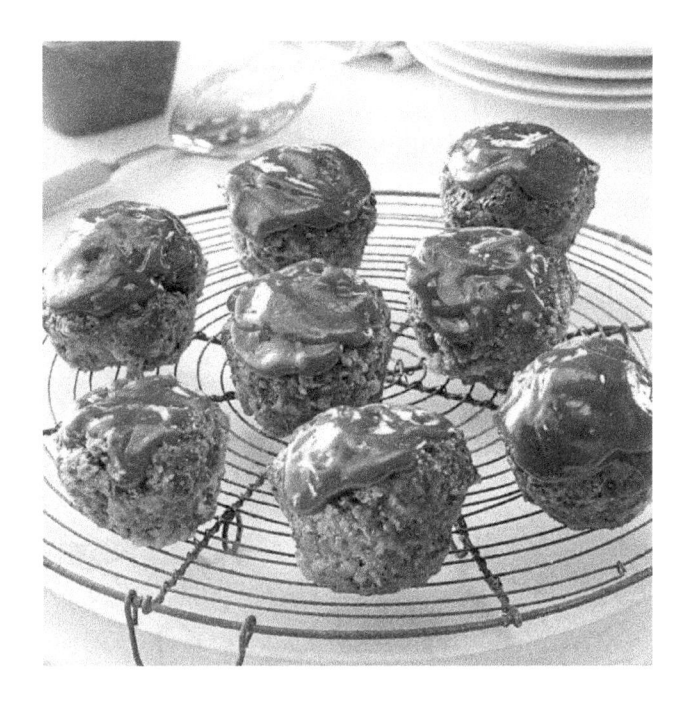

Prep: 20 min. Bake: 30 min.

Ingredients

1. 1 cup ketchup

2. 3 to 4 tablespoons packed brown sugar
3. 1 teaspoon ground mustard
4. 2 large eggs, lightly beaten
5. 4 teaspoons Worcestershire sauce
6. 3 cups Crispix cereal, crushed
7. 3 teaspoons onion powder
8. 1/2 to 1 teaspoon seasoned salt
9. 1/2 teaspoon garlic powder
10. 1/2 teaspoon pepper
11. 3 pounds lean ground beef (90% lean)

INSTRUCTIONS:

- In a large bowl, combine the ketchup, brown sugar and mustard. Remove 1/2 cup for topping; set aside. Add the eggs, Worcestershire sauce, cereal and seasonings to remaining ketchup mixture. Let stand for 5 minutes. Crumble beef over cereal mixture and mix well.

- Press meat mixture into 18 muffin cups (about 1/3 cup each). Bake at 375° for 18-20 minutes. Drizzle with reserved ketchup mixture; bake 10 minutes longer or until meat is no longer pink and a thermometer reads 160°.

- Serve desired number of meat loaves. Cool remaining loaves. Transfer to freezer container; close and freeze for up to 3 months.

- To use frozen meat loaves: Completely thaw in the refrigerator. Place loaves in a greased baking dish. Bake at 350° for 30 minutes or until heated through, or cover and microwave on high for 1 minute or until heated through.

Bacon-Topped Meat Loaf

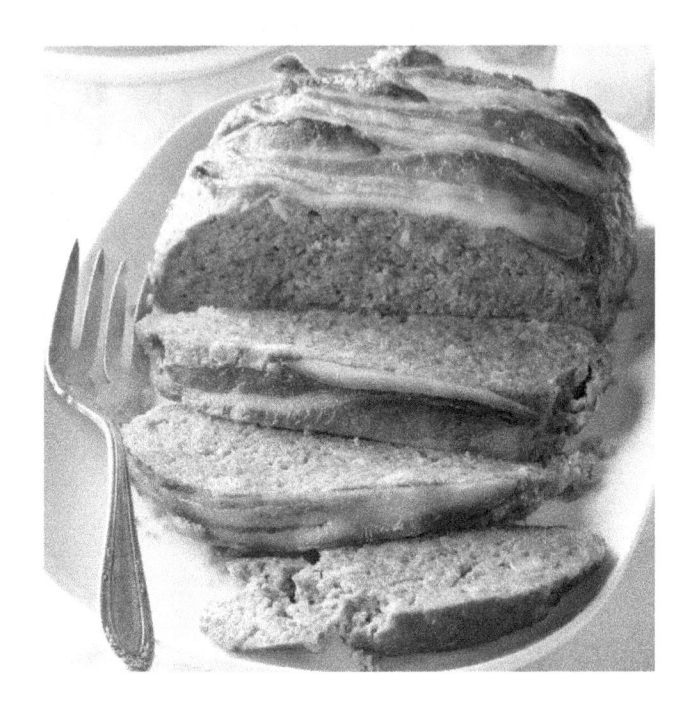

Prep: 10 min. Bake: 70 min. + standing

Ingredients

1. 1/2 cup chili sauce
2. 2 large eggs, lightly beaten
3. 1 tablespoon Worcestershire sauce

4. 1 medium onion, chopped

5. 1 cup shredded cheddar cheese

6. 2/3 cup dry bread crumbs

7. 1/2 teaspoon salt

8. 1/4 teaspoon pepper

9. 2 pounds lean ground beef (90% lean)

10. 2 bacon strips, halved

INSTRUCTIONS:

- In a large bowl, combine the first eight ingredients. Crumble beef over mixture and mix well. Shape into a loaf in an ungreased 13x9-in. baking dish. Top with bacon.

- Bake, uncovered, at 350° for 70-80 minutes or until meat is no longer pink and a thermometer reads 160°. Drain; let stand for 10 minutes before cutting.

Easy Asian Glazed Meatballs

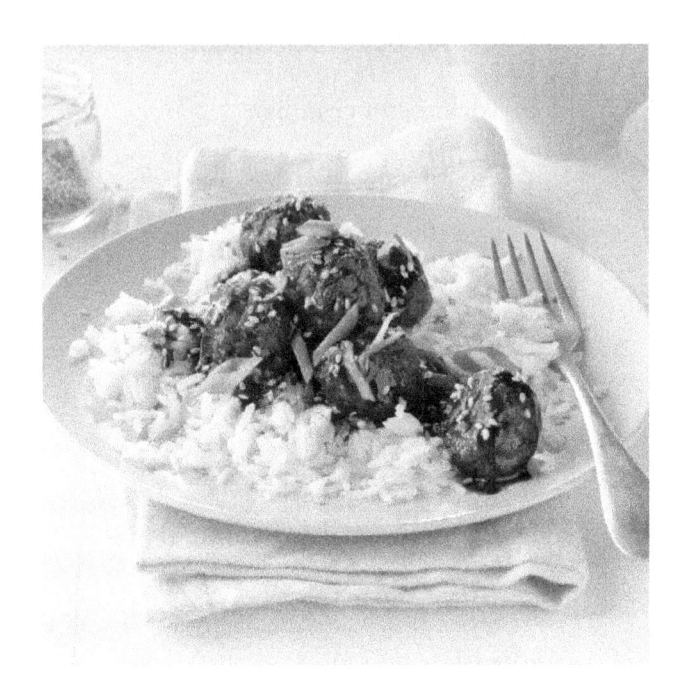

Total Time
Prep/Total Time: 20 min.

Ingredients

1. 1/2 cup hoisin sauce
2. 2 tablespoons rice vinegar
3. 4 teaspoons brown sugar

4. 1 teaspoon garlic powder

5. 1 teaspoon Sriracha chili sauce

6. 1/2 teaspoon ground ginger

7. 1 package (12 ounces) frozen fully cooked homestyle or Italian meatballs, thawed

8. Thinly sliced green onions and toasted sesame

seeds, optional

9. Hot cooked rice

INSTRUCTIONS:

- In a large saucepan, mix the first six ingredients until blended. Add meatballs, stirring to coat; cook, covered, over medium-low heat until heated through, 12-15 minutes, stirring occasionally.

- If desired, sprinkle with green onions and sesame seeds. Serve with rice.

Asian-Style Round Steak

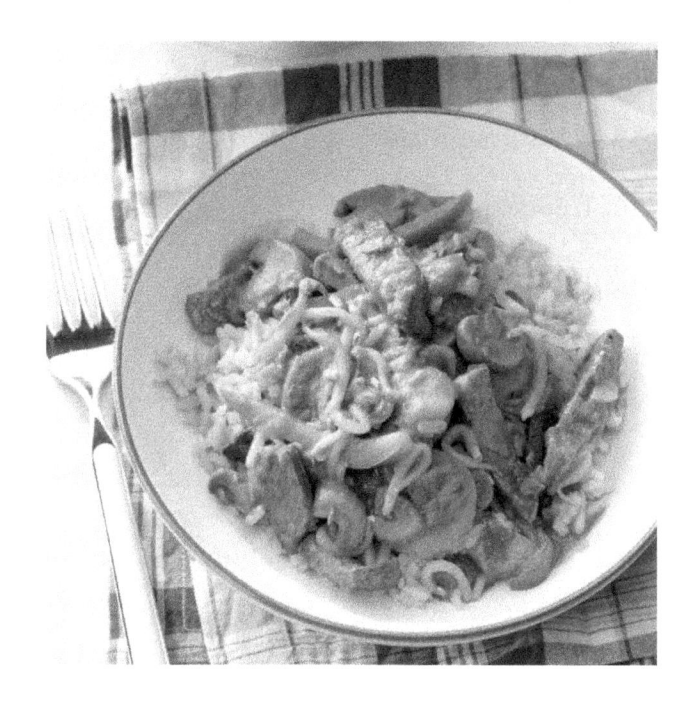

Total Time
Prep: 20 min. Cook: 7 hours

Ingredients

10. 2 pounds beef top round steak, cut into 3-inch strips

11. 2 tablespoons canola oil

12. 3 celery ribs, chopped

13. 1 cup chopped onion

14. 1/4 cup reduced-sodium soy sauce

15. 1 teaspoon sugar

16. 1/2 teaspoon minced garlic

17. 1/4 teaspoon ground ginger

18. 1/4 teaspoon pepper

19. 2 medium green peppers, julienned

20. 1 can (15 ounces) tomato sauce

21. 1 can (14 ounces) bean sprouts, rinsed and drained

22. 1 can (8 ounces) sliced water chestnuts, drained

23. 1 jar (4-1/2 ounces) sliced mushrooms, drained

24. 1 tablespoon cornstarch

25. 1/2 cup cold water

26. Hot cooked rice

27. Minced chives, optional

INSTRUCTIONS:

- In a large skillet, brown meat in oil on all sides. Transfer meat and drippings to a 5-qt. slow cooker. Combine the celery, onion, soy sauce, sugar, garlic, ginger and pepper; pour over meat. Cover and cook on low for 5-1/2 to 6 hours or until meat is tender.

- Add the green peppers, tomato sauce, bean sprouts, water chestnuts and mushrooms; cover and cook on low 1 hour longer.

- Combine cornstarch and water until smooth; stir into beef mixture. Cover and cook on high for 30 minutes or until sauce is thickened. Serve with rice; if desired, sprinkle with chives.

Meat Loaf Dinner

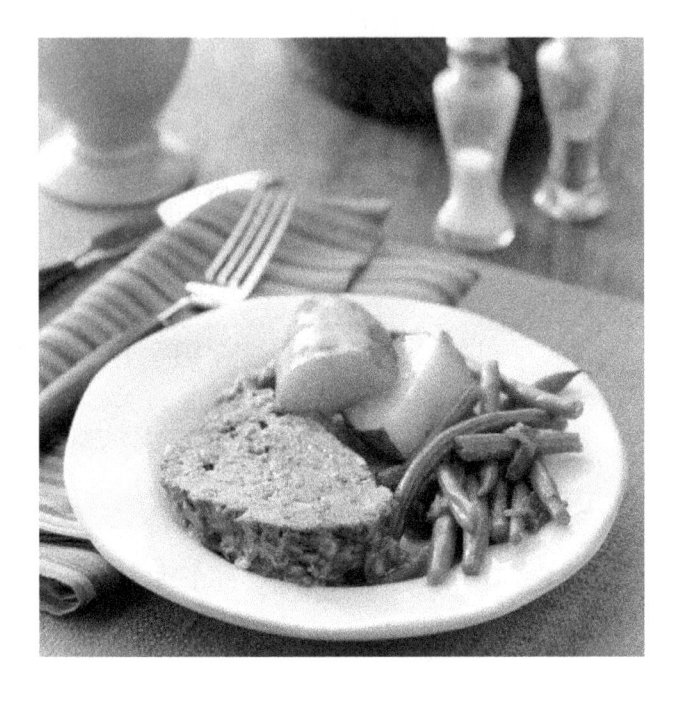

Prep: 15 min. Bake: 2 hours

Ingredients

1. 1 egg
2. 1/2 cup seasoned bread crumbs
3. 1/4 cup chopped onion

4. 1/2 teaspoon seasoned salt

5. 2 pounds lean ground beef

6. 4 medium potatoes, quartered

7. 1/2 pound fresh or frozen cut green beans

8. 1 can (14-1/2 ounces) stewed tomatoes

INSTRUCTIONS:

- In a large bowl, combine the first four ingredients. Crumble beef over mixture and mix well. Shape into a loaf in a greased roasting pan. Arrange potatoes and green beans around loaf. Pour tomatoes over all.

- Cover and bake at 350°: for 2 hours or until the meat is no longer pink and a thermometer reads 160°.

Pressure Cooker Mushroom Pot Roast

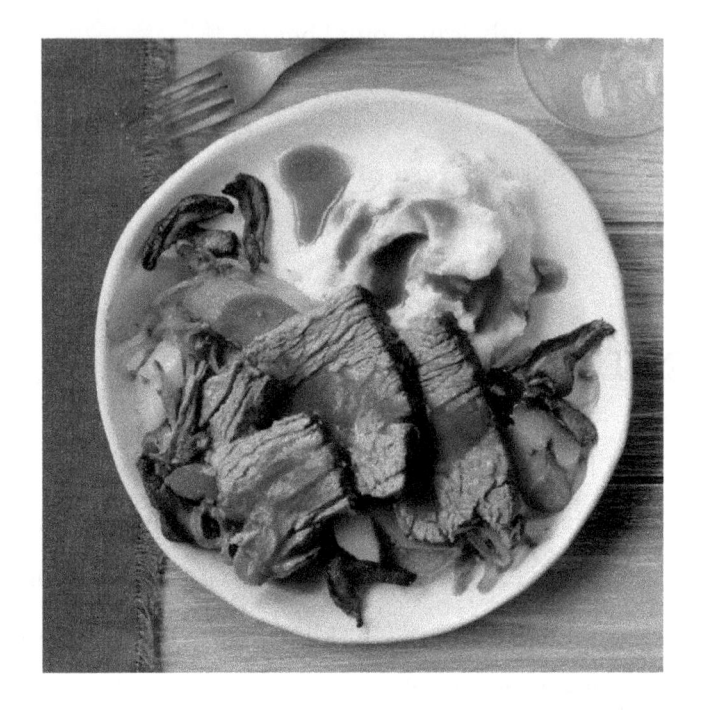

Prep: 25 min. Cook: 65 min. + releasing

Ingredients

1. 1 boneless beef chuck roast (3 to 4 pounds)

2. 1/2 teaspoon salt

3. 1/4 teaspoon pepper

4. 1 tablespoon canola oil

5. 1-1/2 cups dry red wine or reduced-sodium beef broth

6. 1-1/2 pounds sliced fresh shiitake mushrooms

7. 2-1/2 cups thinly sliced onions

8. 1-1/2 cups reduced-sodium beef broth

9. 1 can (8 ounces) tomato sauce

10. 3/4 cup chopped peeled parsnips

11. 3/4 cup chopped celery

12. 3/4 cup chopped carrots

13. 8 garlic cloves, minced

14. 2 bay leaves

15. 1-1/2 teaspoons dried thyme

16. 1 teaspoon chili powder

17. 1/4 cup cornstarch

18. 1/4 cup water

19. Mashed potatoes

INSTRUCTIONS:

- Halve roast; sprinkle with salt and pepper. Select saute or browning setting on a 6-qt. electric pressure cooker. Adjust for medium heat; add 1-1/2 teaspoons oil. When oil is hot, brown one roast half on all sides. Remove; repeat with remaining beef and 1-1/2 teaspoons oil. Add wine to pressure cooker. Cook 2 minutes, stirring to loosen browned bits from pan. Press cancel. Return beef to pressure cooker.

- Add mushrooms, onions, broth, tomato sauce, parsnips, celery, carrots, garlic, bay leaves, thyme and chili powder. Lock lid; close pressure-release valve. Adjust to pressure-cook on high for 60 minutes. Let pressure release naturally for 10 minutes; quick-release any remaining pressure. A thermometer inserted in beef should read at least 160°.

- Remove meat and vegetables to a serving platter; keep warm. Discard bay leaves. Skim fat from cooking juices; transfer back to pressure cooker. In a

- small bowl, mix cornstarch and water until smooth; stir into cooking juices. Select saute setting and adjust for low heat. Simmer, stirring constantly, until thickened, 1-2 minutes. Serve with mashed potatoes, meat and vegetables.

- Freeze option: Place roast and vegetables in freezer containers; top with cooking juices. Cool and freeze. To use, partially thaw in refrigerator overnight. Heat through in a covered saucepan, stirring gently and adding a little broth if necessary.

CHEWY GRANOLA BAR RECIPE

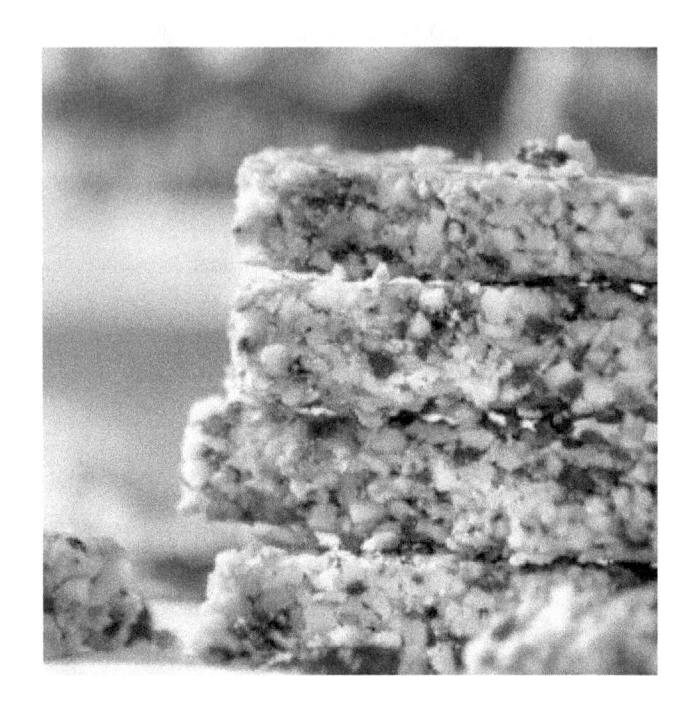

MACROS PER SERVING:

Cal 180, Fat 17g, Protein 4g, Carbs 2g

Prep time: 10 mins
Cook time: 25 mins

Ingredients

1. 1/2 cups sliced almonds
2. 1/2 cup flaked coconut (unsweetened)
3. 1/2 cup pecans
4. 1/2 cup sunflower seeds
5. 1/2 cup dried, unsweetened cranberries (chopped)
6. 1/2 cup butter
7. 1/2 cup So Nourished powdered erythritol
8. 1/2 tsp vanilla extract
9. 1 pinch salt

Method

- Preheat the oven to 300°F and line a square baking dish with parchment.
- Combine the almonds, coconut, pecans, and sunflower seeds in a food processor.

- Pulse the mixture until finely chopped and crumb-like, like granola.

- Pour the mixture into a bowl and stir in the cranberries and a pinch of salt.

- Melt the butter in a saucepan over low heat then whisk in the erythritol and vanilla extract.

- Pour the mixture over the granola and stir until well combined.

- Press the mixture into the prepared dish, compacting it as much as possible, and bake for 25 minutes.

- Cool the mixture in the pan completely then remove and cut into 16 bars.

BLUEBERRY COCONUT PORRIDGE

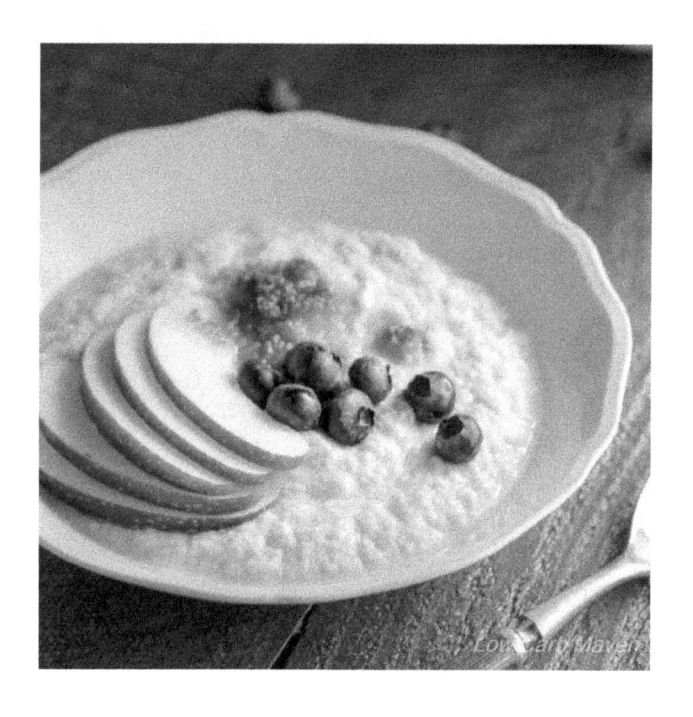

MACROS PER SERVING:

Cal 405, Fat 34g, Protein 10g, Carbs 8g

Prep Time: 5 mins
Cook Time: 5 mins

Ingredients

1. Porridge
2. 1 cup almond milk
3. 1/4 cup
4. 1 tsp vanilla extract
5. 10 drops liquid stevia
6. 1 pinch salt

Toppings

7. 2 tbsp butter
8. 60 grams blueberries
9. 2 tbsp pumpkin seeds
10. 1 oz. shaved coconut

Method

- Set a cup of almond milk to heat up on a low flame.

- Add in flaxseed, coconut flour, cinnamon and salt. Use a whisk to break up any clumps.

- Heat until slightly bubbling. Add in liquid stevia and vanilla extract.

- When the mixture is as thick as you want it to be, turn off the flame and add in your toppings. We like to add cold butter, fresh or frozen blueberries, pumpkin seeds and shaved coconut!

BLINI STYLE CAVIAR CREPES

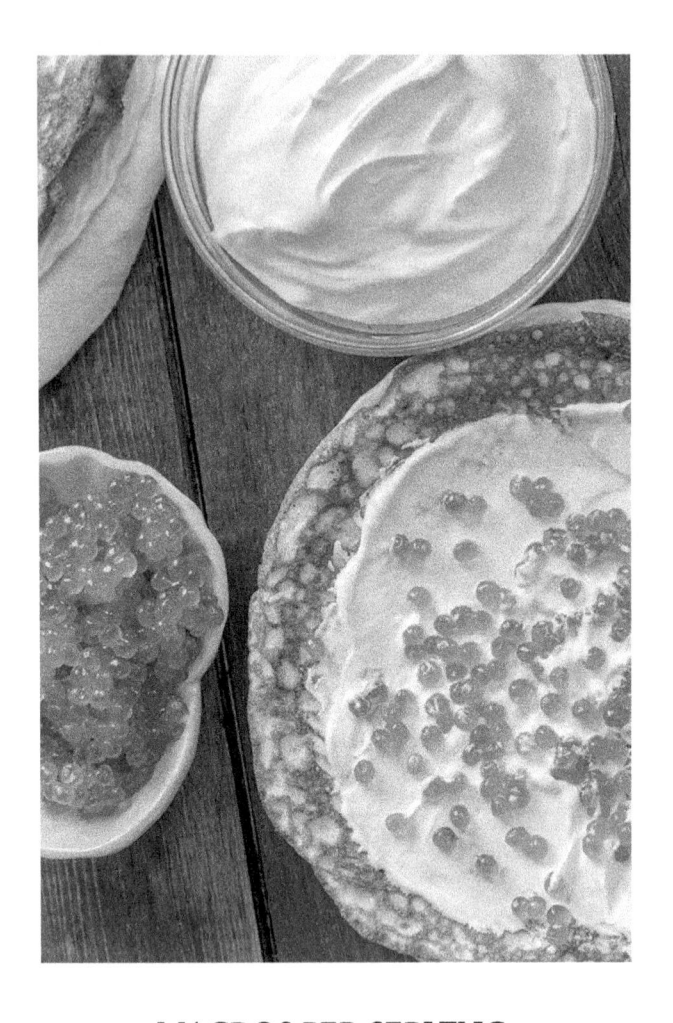

MACROS PER SERVING:

Cal 535, Fat 38g, Protein 40g, Carbs 4g

Prep time: 10 mins
Cook time: 10 mins

Ingredients

Blini

1. 2 oz. cream cheese
2. 2 large eggs
3. 1/2 tsp baking powder
4. 1 pinch sea salt

Filling

5. 1/2 cup sour cream
6. 3/4 cup wild Alaskan salmon caviar

Method

- Prepare the blini style crepes by combining all the ingredients in a food processor or blender and blending until smooth.

- Heat up a small skillet with a bit of butter on medium heat. Let it heat up fully! Ladle a little less than 1/4 cup of batter in at a time and swirl the contents around to spread it evenly.

- Cook until the edges start to peel away from the skillet and bubbles have formed on top. This should take about 2-3 minutes per crepe.

- Flip and cook for another minute. Repeat with all the batter. This recipe should make 4 medium sized crepes.

- Once the batter has cooked and the crepes are ready, spoon 2 tablespoons of sour cream onto each, followed by 2-3 tablespoons of wild Alaskan salmon caviar. Roll each up and enjoy!

CHICKEN CAPRESE ZOODLE BOWLS

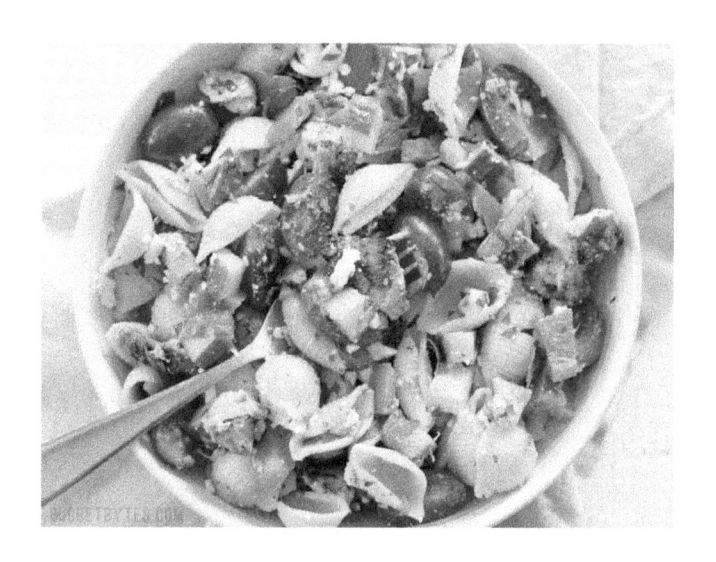

Chicken Caprese Zoodle Bowls are the perfect light, fresh, summer meal. Made with spiralized zucchini and fresh tomatoes, they're gluten free and delicious!

MACROS PER SERVING:

Calories 342, Fat 17g, Carbohydrates 14g, Protein 34g

Prep time: 5 mins
Cook time: 20 mins

Ingredients

1. 1 lb boneless skinless chicken breast cleaned and pounded- thin
2. 2 large zucchini
3. 1 c cherry tomatoes halved
4. ½ c mini mozzarella balls halved
5. ¼ c chopped basil separated
6. 2 tablespoons olive oil separated
7. 2 tablespoons balsamic vinegar for dressing
8. Sea salt + pepper

Method

- In a large skillet heat 1 tbsp olive oil. Cook chicken 7-8 minutes on each side until browned.

- Spiralize 2 large zucchini, Chop tomatoes, mozzarella, and basil.

- In a bowl combine zoodles, cherry tomatoes, mozzarella balls, basil, olive oil, salt + pepper. Toss until everything is thoroughly coated.

- Plate the zoodles and top with cooked chicken and balsamic glaze

LOW CARB PIZZA CHICKEN SKILLET

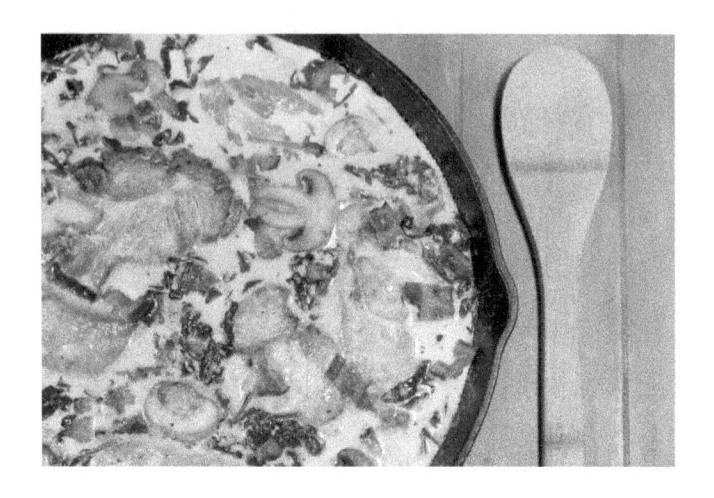

An easy low carb chicken skillet recipe that's so simple to prepare. Just brown boneless skinless chicken meat and smother with pizza toppings.

MACROS PER SERVING:

Cal 337, Fat 18g, Carbs 3g, Protein 37g

Prep time: 5 mins
Cook time: 15 mins

Ingredients

1. 2 tablespoons avocado oil or olive oil

   1.5 pounds skinless/boneless chicken pieces about 5 thighs

2. 1/4 teaspoon salt sprinkle to taste

3. 1/8 teaspoon pepper sprinkle to taste

4. 2 cloves garlic minced

5. 1 cup low carb pizza sauce or marinara sauce

6. 5 slices mozzarella cheese

7. 1 ounce pepperoni slices

Method

- Heat oil in skillet over medium high heat. Season chicken with salt and pepper.

- Add seasoned chicken and garlic to skillet. Cook chicken until browned.

- Pour pizza or marinara sauce on top. Allow to simmer until sauce is heated.

- Top each piece of chicken with a slice of mozzarella cheese and pieces of

pepperoni.

- Cover skillet until cheese is melted or place skillet under broiler to melt cheese and serve immediately.

TEQUILA LIME CHICKEN

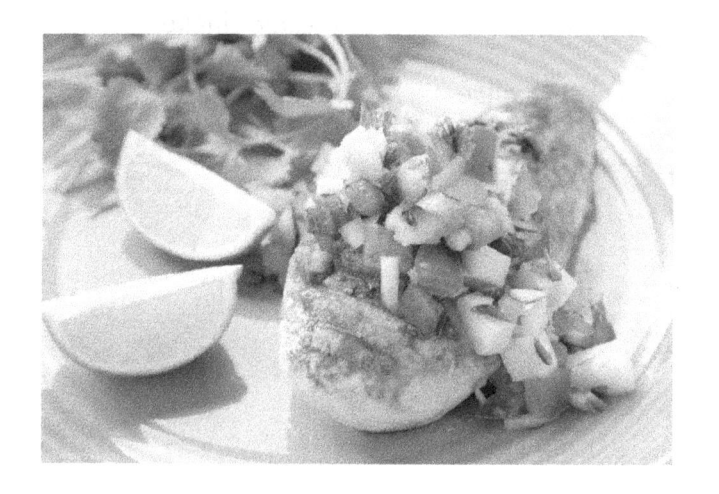

Tequila Lime Chicken is packed with vibrant flavors and cooks in under 30 min- A fun and festive Mexican-style dish perfect for friday night dinner parties and week-night meals alike!

MACROS PER SERVING:

Cal 488, Fat 41.1g , Carbs 2.7g, Protein 16.1g

Prep time: 15 mins
Cook time: 7 mins

Ingredients

1. 2 skinless free-range organic chicken breasts
2. 1 tbsp olive oil, for grilling
3. For the marinade:
4. 1 tbsp extravirgin olive oil
5. ¼ cup good-quality gold tequila
6. zest of 2 limes
7. 1 tsp light honey
8. 1 tbsp hot or mild paprika powder
9. 1 thai red chilli, finely minced
10. 1 garlic clove, finely minced
11. a generous pinch of sea salt and cayenne pepper

To serve:

12. ½ cup pinepple salsa
13. lime wedges
14. fresh cilantro, chopped

Method

- Whisk all the marinade ingredients together in a bowl. Add the chicken breasts into the marinade, and stir well to combine.

- Divide the chicken into two zip-log bags, and pour half the marinade on each breast. Close the bags and marinate in the fridge for 15 minutes but best for 2 hours.

- Drizzle with oil a grill pan, and heat until medium-high heat.

- Place the chicken breasts on the grill and spoon any remaining marinade from the bag over top. Grill, covered, for 4 minutes one one side. Turn the breast and cook a further 5 mins.

- Serve immediately with lime wedges on the side, and top with fresh cilantro and a spoonful of pineapple salsa

CHICKEN AND CAULIFLOWER SKILLET

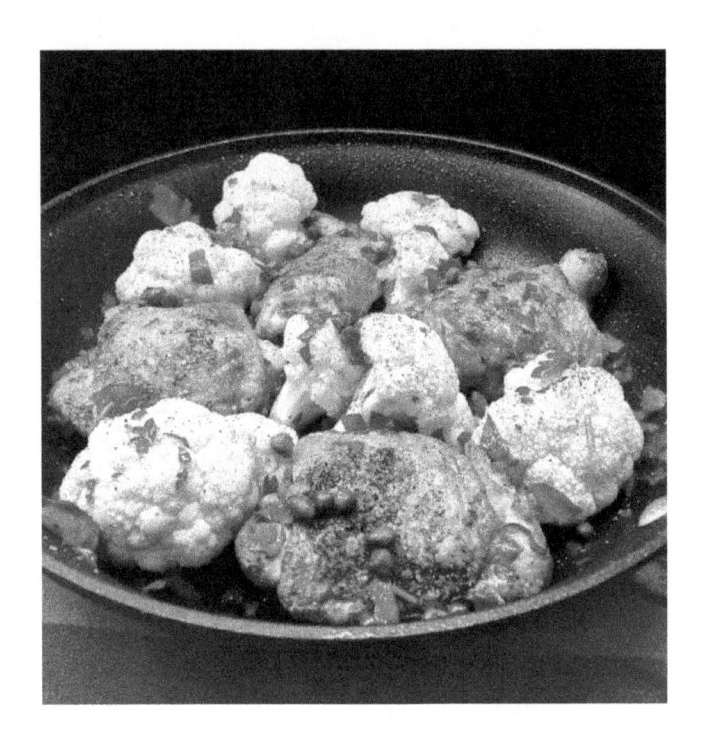

Healthy Chicken Cauliflower Skillet features sauteed chicken baked with yummy cauliflower, covered with a sherry vinegar sauce, parsley, and capers.

MACROS PER SERVING:

Cal 150, Fat 2.5g, Carbs 13g, Protein 20g.

Prep time: 10 mins
Cook time: 30 mins

Ingredients

1. 4 chicken thighs bone-in, skin-on
2. 1 Tbsp olive oil
3. 1 head cauliflower broken up into large florets
4. 1/4 cup fresh parsley chopped
5. 3 Tbsp sherry vinegar
6. 2 Tbsp capers

Method

- Preheat your oven to 450 degrees.
- Heat a large oven-proof skillet over medium-high heat. Add the olive oil. Season the chicken thighs with salt and pepper, place in

the skillet skin side down. Cook the chicken for 5-6 minutes, or until the skin is golden brown. Turn the chicken over and cook for an additional 3-4 minutes.

- Remove from the heat, arrange the cauliflower florets around the chicken and make sure to coat them with the pan juices. Season lightly with salt and pepper.

- Put the skillet in the oven and cook for about 20 minutes, or until the chicken is done and the cauliflower is crisp-tender.

- Carefully remove the pan from the oven, add the sherry vinegar, and sprinkle the parsley and capers over the chicken. Serve immediately. Enjoy!

BROILED CHICKEN THIGHS WITH ARTICHOKES AND GARLIC

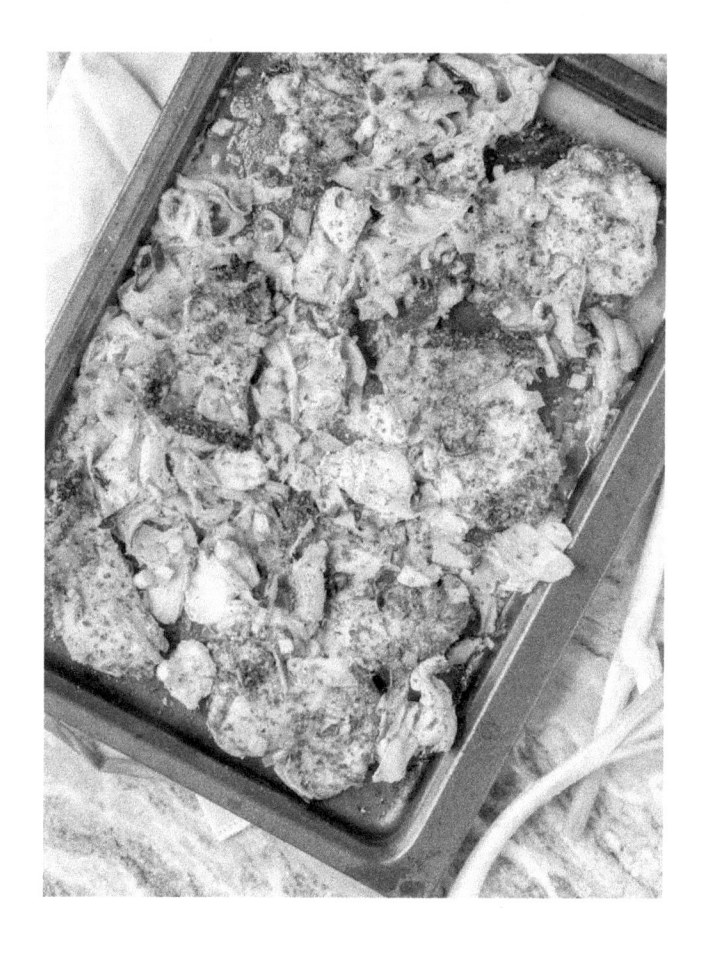

Only 4 key ingredients needed for these low fuss, minimal clean up 30 minute artichoke and garlic broiled chicken thighs. A classic go to weeknight dinner recipe. Healthy and delicious. Gluten Free and Dairy Free.

MACROS PER SERVING:

Cal 261, Fat 10g, Carbs 5g, Protein 33g

Prep time: 10 mins
Cook time: 20 mins

Ingredients

1. 1.5 pounds boneless skinless chicken thighs 6
2. 1-2 jars artichoke hearts (10 ounce jars)
3. 2 tablespoons dried oregano
4. 2 tablespoons minced garlic
5. salt and pepper to taste

Method

- Mix chicken thighs and artichoke hearts (including liquid) in a large bowl. Allow to marinate for 20-30 minutes (optional).
- Drain the liquid.
- Add oregano, minced garlic, salt and pepper and mix.
- Broil on high for 20-25 minutes or until chicken is cooked through. (Broil on the second or third rack from the top for the first 20 minutes and then place the baking tray on the top oven shelf - closer to the broiler, to get a nice crisp on the chicken for the last 5 minutes)
- Optional: halfway through cooking time you can flip over the chicken thighs, if you like.

KEY LIME CHEESECAKE BARS

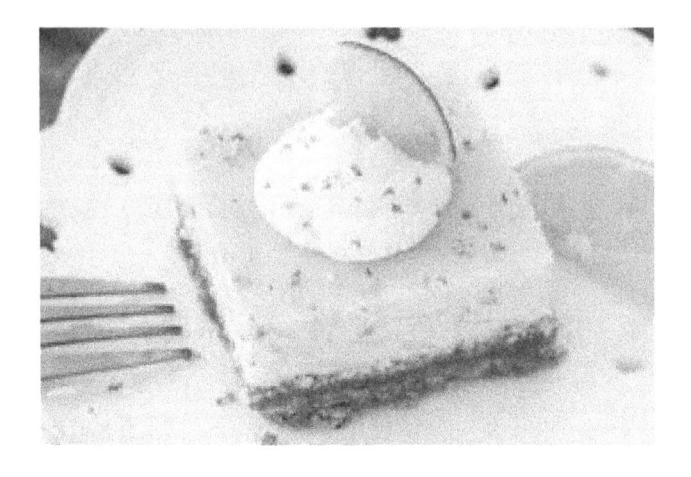

These simple Key Lime Pie Bars have a simple ingredient graham cracker crust with a homemade key lime pie filling on top.

MACROS PER SERVING:

Cal 244, Sugar 9g, Fat 21g, Carbs 11g, Protein 5g

Prep time: 1 hr 15 mins
Cook time: 15 mins

Ingredients

For the crust

1. 1/2 cups graham cracker crumbs
2. 1/3 cup granulated sugar
3. 1/3 cup butter, melted
4. For the filling
5. 14 ounce can sweetened condensed milk
6. 1/4 cup sour cream
7. 2 large egg yolks
8. 1/2 cup key lime juice
9. zest of 1 lime
10. fresh whipped cream , for topping, optional

Method

For the Crust:

- For the crust, Combine the graham cracker crumbs, sugar, and butter and press into an 8" square baking pan. Bake at 350 degrees F for 5 minutes.

For the Filling:

- Make the filling by combining all ingredients. Pour the filling into the warm crust and bake for 8-12 minutes or until the center is just set. Allow to cool completely. Refrigerate for several hours before serving. Top with fresh whipped cream, if desired.

KETO PEPPERMINT CHOCOLATE

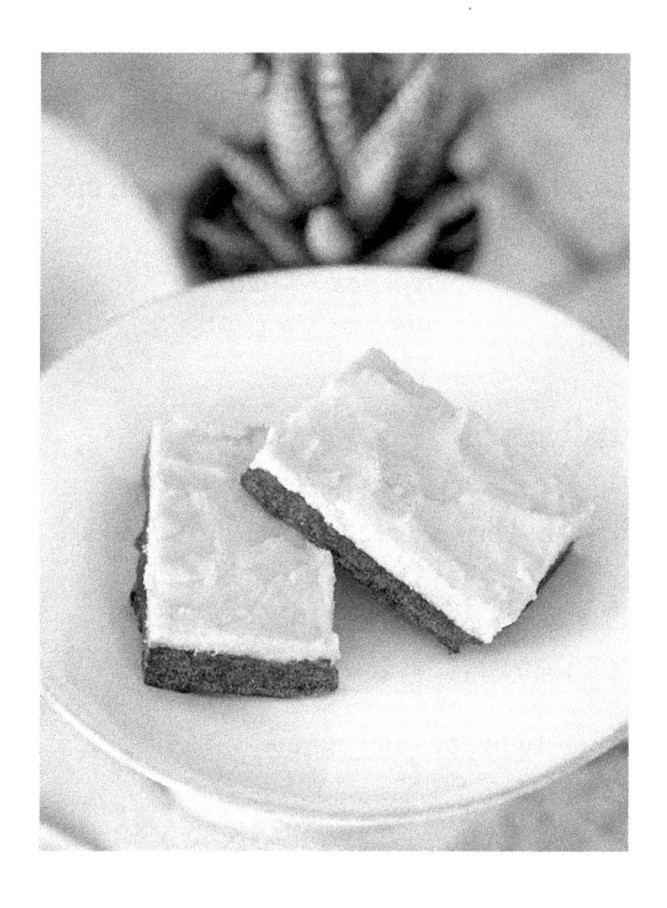

Ring in the holiday season with this low-carb chocolate peppermint cheesecake mousse. It's an easy sugar free dessert that's ready in a snap, but it looks and tastes elegant enough to serve your guests.

MACROS PER SERVING:

Cal 39, Fat: 4.3 g, Carbs: 0.5 g, Protein: 0.5 g

Prep time: 5 mins
Cook time: 10 mins

Ingredients

1. 6 oz Unsweetened Chocolate (6 squares)
2. 3/4 cup heavy cream
3. 1 stick butter
4. 1 tsp peppermint extract
5. 2 tbsp Stevia
6. 1 tbsps vanilla extract optional
7. Dash of sea salt optional
8. Peppermint Fudge

Method

- Add the chocolate and butter together and melt them over low heat.

- When the chocolate mixture is completely melted, remove from the heat and blend with the vanilla, heavy cream, stevia, and peppermint. Add some salt if necessary.

- Mix the ingredients thoroughly until homogeneous. Gently spread the mix on a non-stick pan.

- Leave in the freezer for 3-4 hours. Slice the chilled chocolate fudge into 50-70 bite-sized cubes. The amount may depend on the size of the pan and the cubes themselves. Store in the freezer until ready to serve. Best enjoyed cold.

LOW CARB LEMON CHEESECAKE

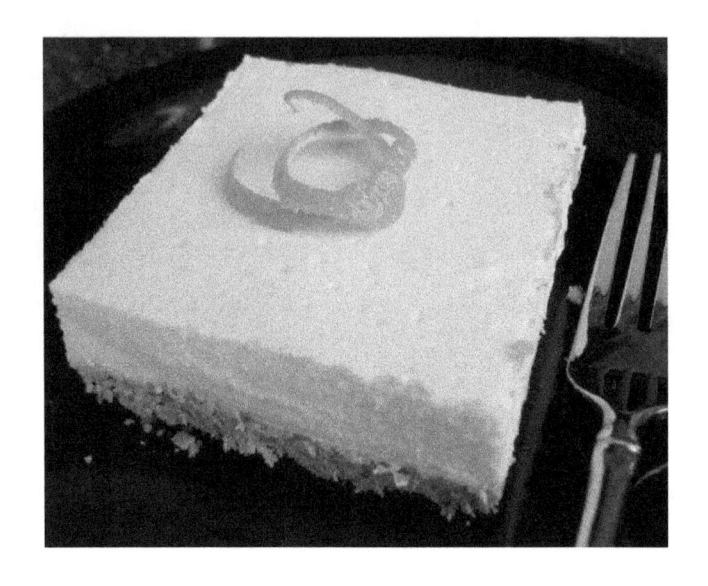

Zingy and refreshing, this lemon low carb cheesecake is a heavenly creamy highlight to any meal. Your family will never guess it's sugar free! Keto, gluten free and diabetic-friendly.

MACROS PER SERVING:

Cal 263, Fat 24.9g, Carbs 5.8g, Protein 7g

Prep time: 10 mins
Cook time: 20 mins

Ingredients

For the base

1. 150 g / 1 1/2 cup almond flour or ground almonds
2. 70 g / 3/4 cup desiccated coconut unsweetened
3. 1 egg large
4. For the filling
5. 300 g / 10.5 oz cream cheese
6. 300 g / 10.5 oz sour cream
7. 1 lemon, zest and juice
8. 2 tbsp powdered sweetener (or more, to taste)
9. 12 g / 1 pack gelatine
10. Get Ingredients Powered by Chicory

Method

- Preheat your oven to 180 Celsius / 356 Fahrenheit.

- Line the bottom of a tart/pie dish with baking paper and grease the sides. In a blender or with a hand mixer (use a tall jug), blend the ingredients for the tart base until they resemble sticky crumbles and the coconut is starting to release its oils. Press the dough into a tart or pie dish with your fingers.

- My dish measured 22 cm at the bottom and 26 cm at the top. Bake for around 20 minutes until the tart crust is lightly browned.

- Remove from the oven and let it cool down. Then remove tart base from the pan.

- Mix the cream cheese, sour cream, sweetener, lemon juice and zest in a bowl until smooth.

-

- Dissolve your gelatine according to your manufacturer's instructions and add to the filling mix.

- Blend and fill into the tart base. Cool the tart in the fridge until set, a minimum of 2 hours or overnight. Decorate with more lemon zest or to your liking.

KETO CHOCOLATE CHIP COOKIES

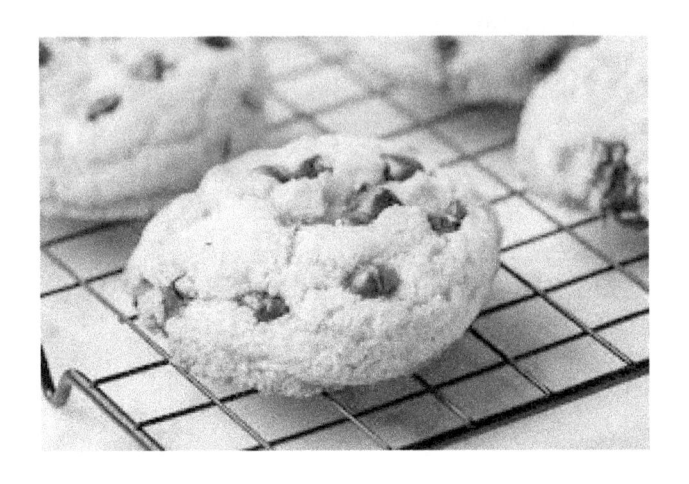

Those living a ketogenic lifestyle get the occasional hankering for this classic every once in a while! The trick in making low carb chocolate chip cookies is to minimize all of the high carb ingredients and maximize the flavor with our ingredients.

MACROS PER SERVING:

Cal 80, Fat 7.1g, Carbs 3.3g, Protein 1.9g

Prep time: 15 mins
Cook time: 10 mins

Ingredients

1. 150g salted butter, softened
2. 80g light brown muscovado sugar
3. 80g granulated sugar
4. 2 tsp vanilla extract
5. 1 large egg
6. 225g plain flour
7. ½ tsp bicarbonate of soda
8. ¼ tsp salt
9. 200g plain chocolate chips or chunks

Method

- Heat the oven to 190C/fan170C/gas 5 and line two baking sheets with non-stick baking paper. Put 150g softened salted butter, 80g light brown muscovado sugar and 80g granulated sugar into a bowl and beat until creamy.

- Beat in 2 tsp vanilla extract and 1 large egg. Sift 225g plain flour, ½ tsp bicarbonate of soda and ¼ tsp salt into the bowl and mix it in with a wooden spoon. Add 200g plain chocolate chips or chunks and stir well.

- Use a teaspoon to make small scoops of the mixture, spacing them well apart on the baking trays. This mixture should make about 30 cookies. Bake for 8–10 mins until they are light brown on the edges and still slightly soft in the centre if you press them. Leave on the tray for a couple of mins to set and then lift onto a cooling rack.

KETO PEANUT BUTTER TAGALONG BARS

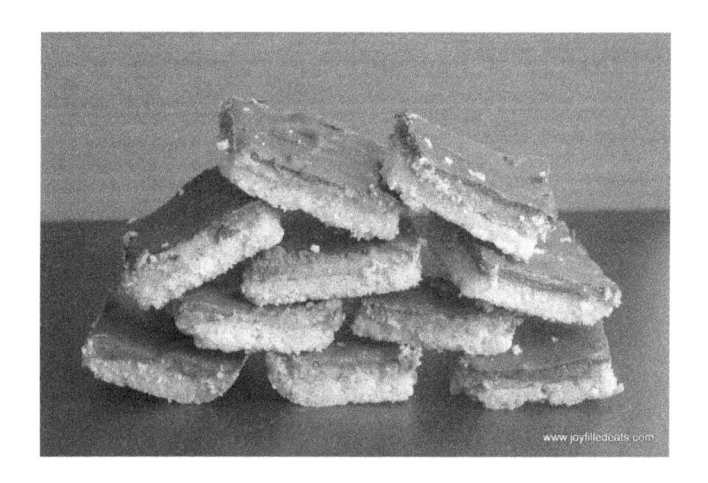

These keto Tagalong cookie bars are far easier to make than individual cookies and they taste just like the original Girl Scout Cookie. Dare I say they taste even better? You won't believe they are low carb and sugar-free.

MACROS PER SERVING:

Cal 214, Fat 19.5g, Carbs 6.51g, Protein 4.68g

Prep time: 15 mins
Cook time: 20 mins

Ingredients

Crust::

1. 1/4 cups almond flour
2. 1/3 cup Swerve Sweetener
3. 1/4 tsp salt
4. 1/4 cup butter chilled and cut into small pieces
5. Peanut Butter Caramel Filling::
6. 2/3 cup creamy peanut butter
7. 1/4 cup butter
8. 1/2 cup powdered Swerve Sweetener
9. 1/4 cup heavy whipping cream
10. 1/2 tsp caramel extract can use vanilla extract

Chocolate Topping:

11. 3 ounces sugar-free dark chocolate such as Lily's, chopped

12. 2 tbsp butter

Method

- Crust:Preheat the oven to 350F. Combine almond flour, butter, sweetener, and salt in a food processor.

- Pulse to combine. Sprinkle the butter over and continue to pulse until the mixture resembles fine crumbs. Press the mixture evenly into the bottom of an 8-inch square pan and bake 15 minutes or until light golden brown. Set aside and let cool.

- Peanut Butter Filling:In a microwave safe bowl, combine the peanut butter and butter and melt on high until it can be stirred to a smooth mixture, about 1 minute. Stir in the powdered sweetener until well combined and then whisk in the cream and the extract. Pour over cooled crust and spread evenly with an offset spatula. Refrigerate until set, about 20 minutes.

Chocolate

- Topping: In a microwave safe bowl, combine the chopped chocolate and the butter. Heat on high in 30 second increments, stirring in between, until smooth. Be careful not to overheat and make your chocolate seize. Spread over the chilled filling. Let set at room temperature for about 1 hour.

KETO SHORTBREAD COOKIES

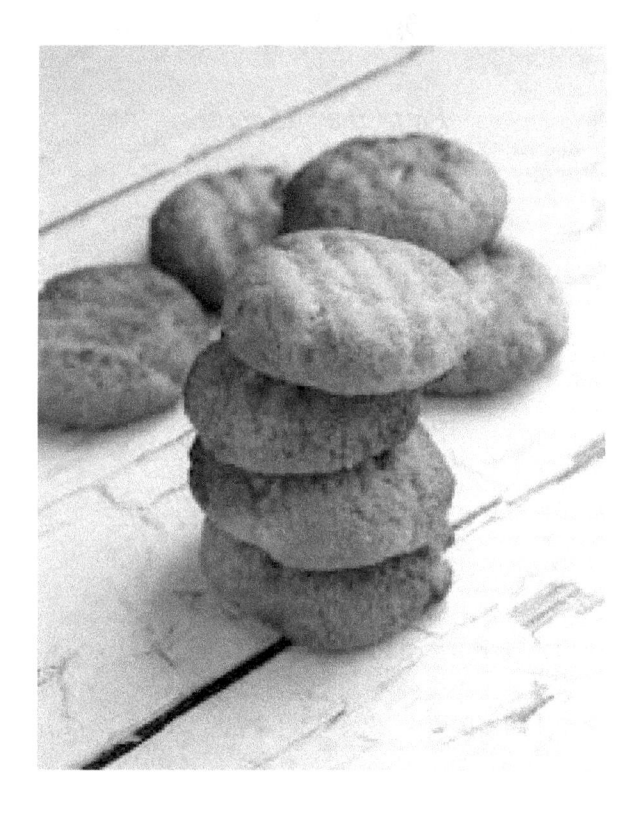

A low carb and entirely sugar free take on classic shortbread biscuits. Keto Shortbread Cookies are light, buttery and crumbly with a deliciously rich coconut butter glaze. Perfect for diabetics, gluten free and ketogenic diets.

MACROS PER SERVING:

Cal 55, Fat 5.3g, Carbs 1.7g, Protein 0.9g

Prep time: 15 mins
Cook time: 6 mins

Ingredients

1. 40 g coconut flour (1/3 cup)
2. 70 g almond flour (2/3 cup)
3. 40 g granulated erythritol (1/4 cup)
4. 8 drops stevia equivalent to 2 tsp of sugar
5. 120 g butter (softened) (1/2 cup)
6. 1 tsp almond or vanilla extract
7. 1/4 tsp baking powder
8. 1/4 tsp xanthan gum (optional)
9. For the glaze:
10. 60 g coconut butter (1/4 cup)
11. 8 drops stevia equivalent to 2 tsp of granulated sweetener

Method

- Preheat the oven to 180 Celsius / 356 Fahrenheit. Mix your dry ingredients.

- Add the softened butter, vanilla/almond extract and stevia and mix until you have a smooth dough.

- Divide the dough into 2 balls and roll out between 2 sheets of baking paper. Place the dough in the fridge for 10 minutes. This will make the dough easier to work with.

- Using a small glass, a cookie cutter, cut your cookies. Place cookies on a baking sheet lined with parchment paper and bake for 6 minutes or until the edges begin to brown. Let the cookies cool completely before adding the glaze.

- Warm the coconut butter in a pot or in the microwave and stir in the sweetener. You can use stevia or powdered erythritol for this.

- Spoon over the cooled cookies and wait for the glaze to set before
- 1) eating or
- 2) storing in an airtight container.

KETO CHOCOLATE MOUSSE

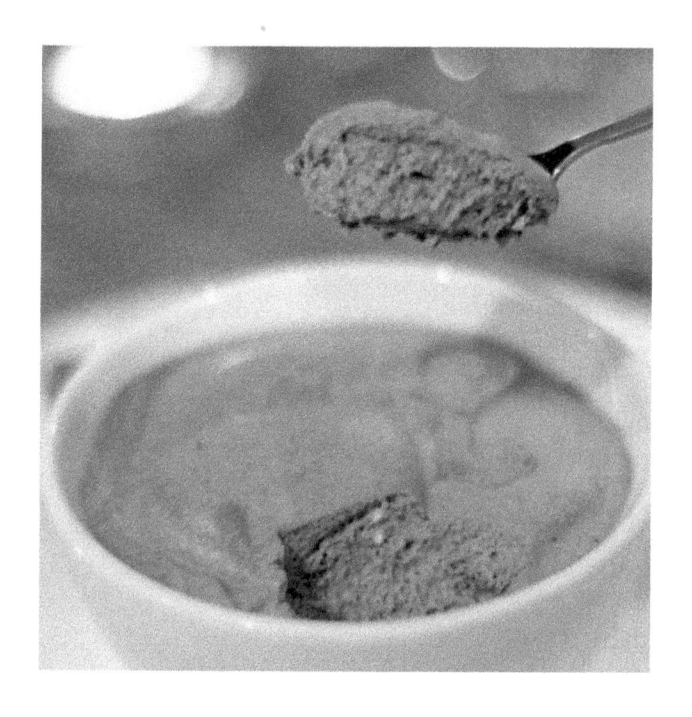

It only takes few minutes to make and tastes delicious on its own, but is also great for a cake filing or frosting.

MACROS PER SERVING:

Cal 239, Carbs 2g, Fat 22g, Protein 3g

Prep time: 5 mins
Cook time: 10 mins

Ingredients

1. 50 grams Dark Chocolate 85%
2. 15 grams Salted Butter or unsalted butter + pinch of salt
3. 1 tbsp Coco Powder
4. 200 ml Whipping Cream
5. Stevia to taste

Method

- Melt the chocolate and butter in the microwave (about 30seconds) and mix together. Whip together cream, cocopowder and stevia.

- Add in the chocolate and butter mix. Whip till soft peaks are formed and put into bowls. Refrigerate for 1 hour at least and serve cold.

KETO CARROT CAKE

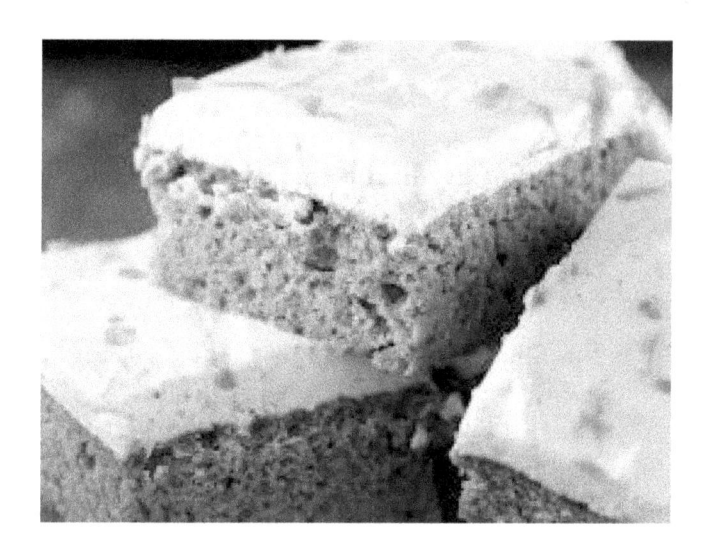

The best keto low carb carrot cake recipe ever! The steps for how to make sugar-free carrot cake are surprisingly easy. So moist and delicious, no one will guess it's gluten-free and sugar-free. Paleo and dairy-free options, too.

MACROS PER SERVING:

Cal 359, Fat 34g, Protein 7.5g

Prep time: 25 mins
Cook time: 30 mins

Ingredients

1. 3/4 cup Erythritol (or coconut sugar for paleo)

2. 3/4 cup Butter (softened; use coconut or ghee for paleo or dairy-free)

3. 1 tbsp Blackstrap molasses (optional)

4. 1 tsp Vanilla extract

5. 1/2 tsp Pineapple extract (optional)

6. 4 large Egg

7. 2 1/2 cup Blanched almond flour

8. 2 tsp Gluten-free baking powder

9. 2 tsp Cinnamon

10. 1/2 tsp Sea salt

11. 2 1/2 cup Carrots (grated, measured loosely packed after grating)

12. 1 1/2 cup Pecans (chopped; divided into 1 cup and 1/2 cup)
13. 2 full recipes Sugar-free cream cheese frosting (double the frosting recipe; for paleo or dairy-free, omit or use a coconut cream based frosting instead)

Method

- Preheat the oven to 350 degrees F (177 degrees C). Line two 9 in (23 cm) round cake pans with parchment paper. (Use springform pans if you have them.)

- Grease the bottom and sides. In a large bowl, cream together the butter and erythritol, until fluffy. Beat in the molasses (if using), vanilla extract, and pineapple extract (if using).

- Beat in the eggs, one at a time. Set aside. In another bowl, mix together the almond flour, baking powder, cinnamon, and sea salt. Stir the dry ingredients into the bowl with the wet ingredients.

- Stir in the grated carrots. Fold 1 cup (340 g) of the chopped pecans, reserving the remaining 1/2 cup (170 g). Transfer the batter evenly among the two prepared baking pans. Bake for 30-35 minutes, until the top is spring-y.

- Let the cakes cool in the pans for 10 minutes, then transfer to a wire rack to cool completely. Meanwhile, make the sugar-free frosting according to the instructions here.

- When the cake has cooled to room temperature, place the bottom layer on a plate or cake stand. Frost, then add the top layer and frost again. Top with the remaining chopped pecans.

FLOURLESS KETO BROWNIES

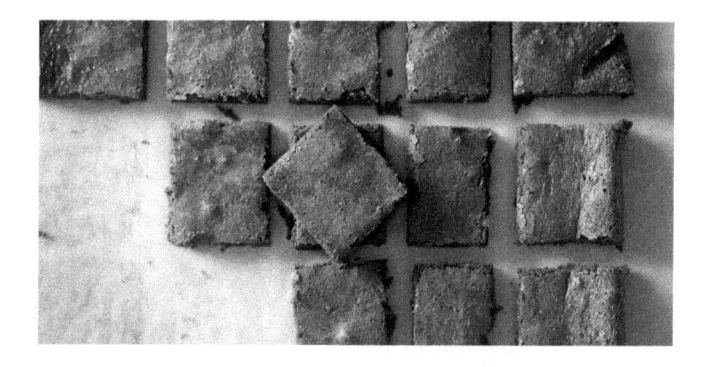

Keto baking can be tough when a recipe calls for ingredients that you may or may not have access to. Sure, if you've been keto for a little while you may have a stockpile of approved flours and additives but what do you do when you run out or if you don't have quite enough almond flour and you are craving a fudgy brownie?

MACROS PER SERVING:

Cal 147, Carbs 5g, Protein 3g, Fat: 15g

Prep time: 5 mins
Cook time: 30 mins

Ingredients

1. 6 tbsp coconut oil
2. 225 grams 100% baking chocolate Can use any baking chocolate of choice
3. 3/4 cup granulated sweetener of choice
4. 2 large eggs To keep it vegan
5. 3 tbsp arrowroot powder
6. 2 tbsp cocoa powder
7. 1/4 cup chocolate chips of choice I used a chopped up Stevia-sweetened milk chocolate bar

Methods

- Preheat the oven to 350 degrees Fahrenheit (175 Celsius). Line an 8 x 8-inch deep pan or brownie pan with parchment paper and set aside.

- In a microwave-safe bowl or stovetop, melt your coconut oil with your baking chocolate of choice. Once smooth and glossy, add all your other ingredients and mix well.

- Pour the brownie batter into the lined pan and bake for 25-30 minutes, and remove once a toothpick comes out 'just' clean from the center. Allow the brownies to cool in the pan completely, before slicing into pieces.

KETO PUMPKIN SPICE MUFFINS WITH ALMOND FLOUR

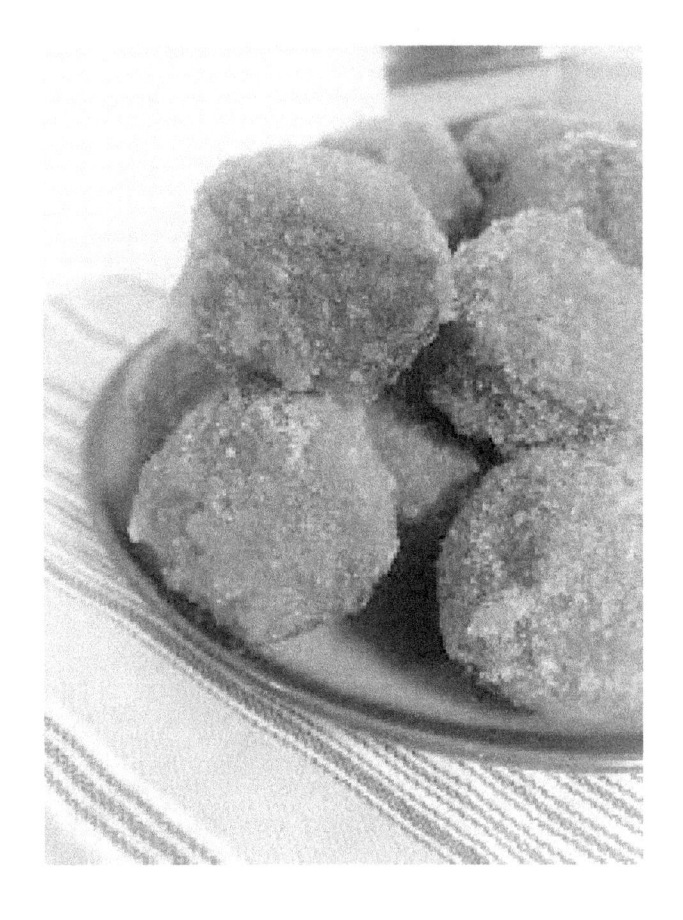

This low carb pumpkin muffins recipe with coconut flour and almond flour is super moist and EASY!

You can also make these keto pumpkin muffins paleo or nut-free if you'd like.

MACROS PER SERVING:

Cal 173 Fat 14g Protein 4g Carbs 7g

Prep time: 10 mins
Cook time: 25 mins

Ingredients

1. 1/2 cup Coconut flour
2. 1/2 cup Blanched almond flour (or sunflower seed meal*)
3. 2/3 cup Erythritol (or any sweetener of choice)
4. 1 tbsp Gluten-free baking powder
5. 1 tbsp Pumpkin pie spice
6. 1/4 tsp Sea salt
7. 4 large Eggs

8. 3/4 cup Pumpkin puree

9. 1/2 cup Ghee (measured solid, then melted; can sub butter or coconut oil)

10. 1 tsp Vanilla extract

11. Pumpkin seeds (for topping - optional)

Method

- Preheat the oven to 350 degrees F (177 degrees C). Line 10 muffin cups with parchment liners.

- In a large bowl, stir together the coconut flour, almond flour, erythritol, baking powder, pumpkin pie spice, and sea salt. Make sure there are no clumps. Stir in the the eggs, pumpkin puree, melted ghee, and vanilla, until completely incorporated.

- Spoon the batter evenly into the muffin cups and smooth the tops. (They should be almost full, not 2/3 or 3/4 full.) If desired, sprinkle pumpkin seeds on top and press gently.

- Bake for about 25 minutes, until an inserted toothpick comes out clean and the muffins are very slightly golden around the edges.

KETO MOULDS BARS

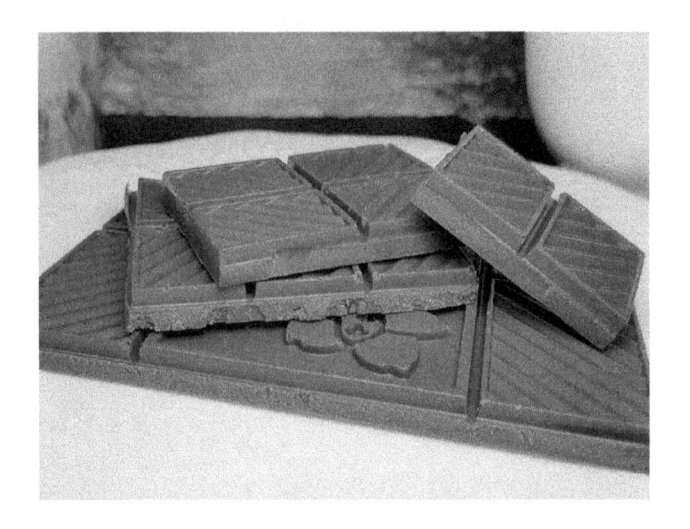

Low carb chocolate is a common request from anyone following a keto diet. Some people wonder if it's possible to have no carb chocolate; unfortunately, the answer is no because even unsweetened 100% cocoa has carbs. And given how bitter unsweetened chocolate is, you need to add some kind of sweetener. To keep it low in carbs, that usually means a sugar free sweetener such as a mixture of stevia and erythritol.

MACROS PER SERVING:

Cal 170, Carbs 3.5g, Protein 3g, Fat 16 g

Prep time: 20 mins
Cook time: 1 hr 40 mins

Ingredients

(makes 12 bars)

Bars:

1. 3 cups shredded unsweetened coconut (225 g/ 8 oz)
2. 1/4 cup powdered Erythritol or Swerve (40 g/ 1.4 oz)
3. 1/2 tsp vanilla powder or 1 tbsp unsweetened vanilla extract
4. 1 cup coconut cream (240 g/ 8.5 oz)
5. 1/4 cup extra virgin coconut oil (55 g/ 1.9 oz)

6. Chocolate coating:

7. 5 oz 85-90% dark chocolate (140 g)

8. 1 1/2 oz cocoa butter or coconut oil (42 g)

Method

- Prepare the coconut cream a day before. If you don't have powdered Erythritol, place some granulated Erythritol in a food processor or a coffee grinder and pulse for a few seconds. Toast the coconut in the oven at 175 °C/ 350 °F for 5-6 minutes.

- Remove from the oven and let it cool down for 10 minutes. Mix the toasted coconut, Erythritol, vanilla, coconut cream and coconut oil. If the mixture is too sticky, place it in the fridge for 10-15 minutes before forming the bars. Using your hands, create 12 bars and place on a tray lined with baking mat or parchment paper. Place in the fridge for 30-60 minutes.

- Meanwhile, melt the dark chocolate and cacao butter in a double boiler or a glass bowl on top of a small saucepan filled with a cup of water over a medium heat. Once completely melted, mix well and turn off the heat. Set aside to cool down before using it for coating.

- Use a wooden stick to hold the coconut bars so you can coat in dark chocolate mixture from all sides. Place on a tray lined with baking mat or parchment paper.

- Drizzle any remaining chocolate on top. Place in the fridge for 30-60 minutes before serving. Keep refrigerated for up to a week, especially if you use coconut oil instead of cocoa butter (coconut oil melts at room temperature).

BAKED LOBSTER TAILS WITH GARLIC BUTTER

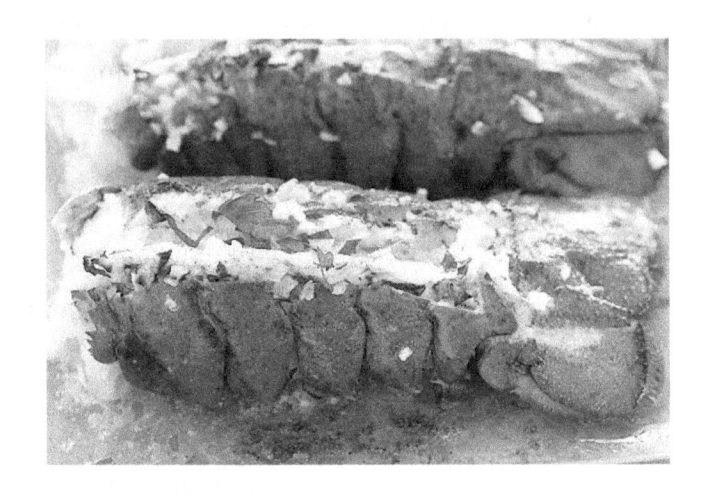

Garlic Butter Lobster Tail - crazy delicious lobster in garlic herb and lemon butter. This lobster tail recipe is so delicious you want it for dinner every day!

MACROS PER SERVING:

Cal 222g, Fat: 14g, Carbs 2g, Protein 21g

Prep time: 10 mins
Cook time: 10 mins

Ingredients

1. 1 lb. shell-on lobster tails (4 lobster tails)
2. cayenne pepper
3. 1/2 stick salted butter, melted (4 tablespoons)
4. 4 cloves garlic, minced
5. 1 tablespoon chopped Italian parsley leaves
6. 1 teaspoon lemon juice
7. lemon slices

Method

- Turn on the broiler on your oven.
- Thaw the lobster tails if they are frozen. Using a pair of kitchen scissors, cut through the top part of the lobster shell, towards the tail. Cut again to a one-inch rectangle shape.

- Remove the lobster shell to expose the lobster meat. Arrange the lobsters on a baking sheet or tray. Add a dash of cayenne pepper on the lobster flesh.

- Melt the butter in a microwave, for about 30 seconds. Add the garlic, parsley and lemon juice to the melted butter. Stir to mix well.

- Drizzle and spread the garlic butter mixture on the lobster. Save some for dipping.

- Broil the lobster tails in the oven for about 5-8minutes, or until the lobster meat turns opaque and cooked through. Serve immediately with the remaining garlic butter and lemon slices.

SUMMER BERRY AND BURRATA SALAD

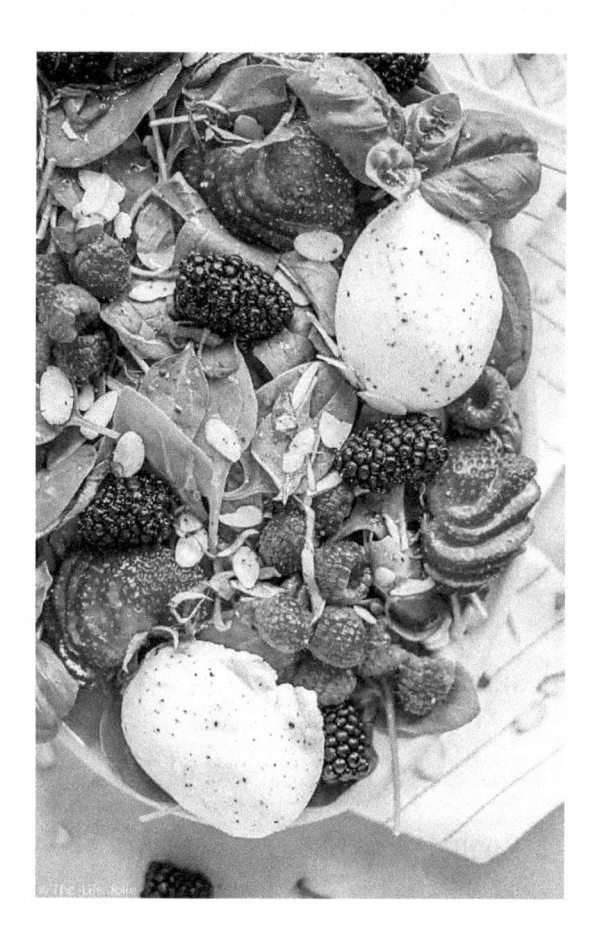

Summer Berry and Burrata Salad is a healthy and delicious recipe. It's easy to make with baby spinach, berries, sliced almonds and creamy Burrata cheese with a homemade honey vinaigrette. This makes a festive side for entertaining guests or a great main dish on a hot summer night when you don't want to cook!

MACROS PER SERVING:

Cal 241, Carbs 7g, Fat 17g, Protein 15 g

Pre time: 10 mins
Cook time: 10 mins

Ingredients

For the salad:

1. 1 5oz. container for baby spinach, washed
2. 1 handful of raspberries, washed
3. 1 handful of blackberries, washed
4. A couple of strawberries
5. 1 handful of sliced almonds

6. A few leaves of sweet basil, cut into a chiffonade
7. 2-3 balls for Burrata cheese
8. For the dressing:
9. 3 Tbsp. extra virgin olive oil
10. 1 1/2 Tbsp. white wine vinegar
11. 1 tsp. honey
12. Salt and pepper to taste

<u>Method</u>

For the salad:

- In a deep bowl, mix the first six ingredients.
- Toss with the dressing until they are evenly coated.
- Place the salad into your serving dish and top with the balls of Burrata and a bit of fresh cracked pepper.

Enjoy!

For the dressing:

- Whisk all ingredients until well combined.

NOTES

To chiffonade the basil, stack the leaves on top of each other and toll them. Then cut the roll (as you would cinnamon buns). You can easily double or triple this recipe for a crown. If Burrata is not available, fresh mozzarella is a good replacement and this also tastes great with crumbly blue cheese. You could easily top this with chicken or shrimp for a more filling entree.

CHICKEN CAPRESE ZOODLE BOWLS

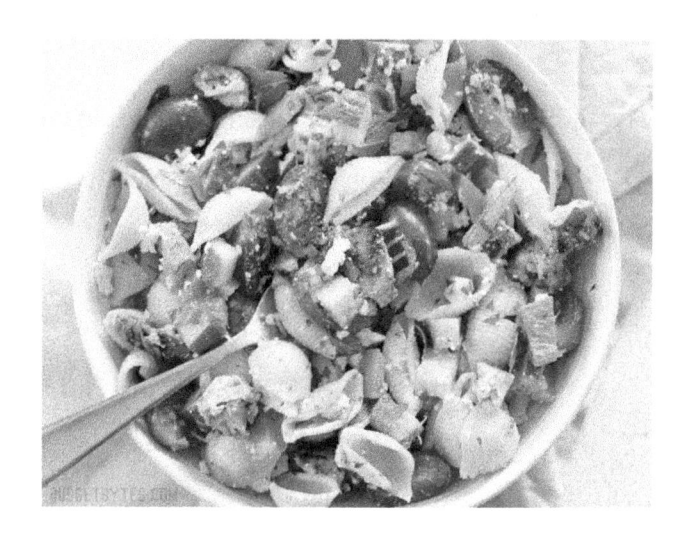

Chicken Caprese Zoodle Bowls are the perfect light, fresh, summer meal. Made with spiralized zucchini and fresh tomatoes, they're gluten free and delicious!

MACROS PER SERVING:

Cal 342, Fat 17g, Carbs 14g, Protein 34g

Prep time: 5 minutes
Cook time: 20 minutes

Ingredients

1. 1 lb boneless skinless chicken breast cleaned and pounded- thin
2. 2 large zucchini
3. 1 c cherry tomatoes halved
4. ½ c mini mozzarella balls halved
5. ¼ c chopped basil separated
6. 2 tablespoons olive oil separated
7. 2 tablespoons balsamic vinegar for dressing
8. Sea salt + pepper

Method

- In a large skillet heat 1 tbsp olive oil. Cook chicken 7-8 minutes on each side until browned.

- Spiralize 2 large zucchini, Chop tomatoes, mozzarella, and basil.

- In a bowl combine zoodles, cherry tomatoes, mozzarella balls, basil, olive oil, salt + pepper. Toss until everything is thoroughly coated.

- Plate the zoodles and top with cooked chicken and balsamic glaze

LOW CARB PIZZA CHICKEN SKILLET

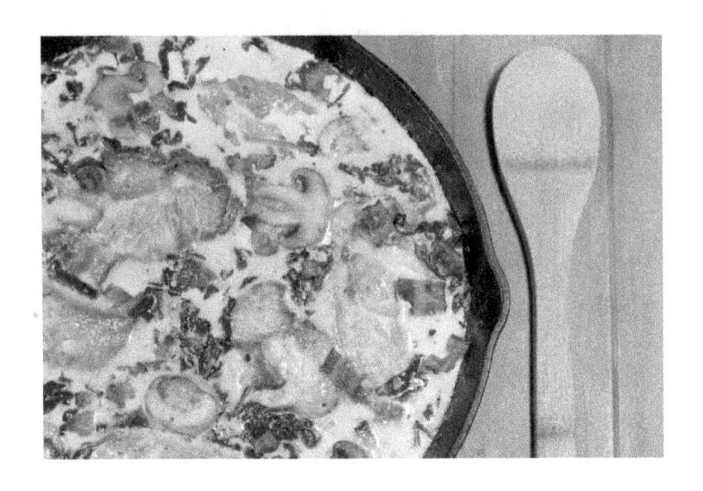

An easy low carb chicken skillet recipe that's so simple to prepare. Just brown boneless skinless chicken meat and smother with pizza toppings.

MACROS PER SERVING:

Cal 337, Fat 18g, Carbs 3g, Protein 37g

Prep time: 5 mins
Cook time: 15 mins

Ingredients

1. 2 tablespoons avocado oil or olive oil

1.5 pounds skinless/boneless chicken pieces about 5 thighs

2. 1/4 teaspoon salt sprinkle to taste

3. 1/8 teaspoon pepper sprinkle to taste

4. 2 cloves garlic minced

5. 1 cup low carb pizza sauce or marinara sauce

6. 5 slices mozzarella cheese

7. 1 ounce pepperoni slices

Method

- Heat oil in skillet over medium high heat. Season chicken with salt and pepper.

- Add seasoned chicken and garlic to skillet. Cook chicken until browned.

- Pour pizza or marinara sauce on top. Allow to simmer until sauce is heated.

- Top each piece of chicken with a slice of mozzarella cheese and pieces of

pepperoni.

- Cover skillet until cheese is melted or place skillet under broiler to melt cheese and serve immediately.

GREEK HERBED LAMB

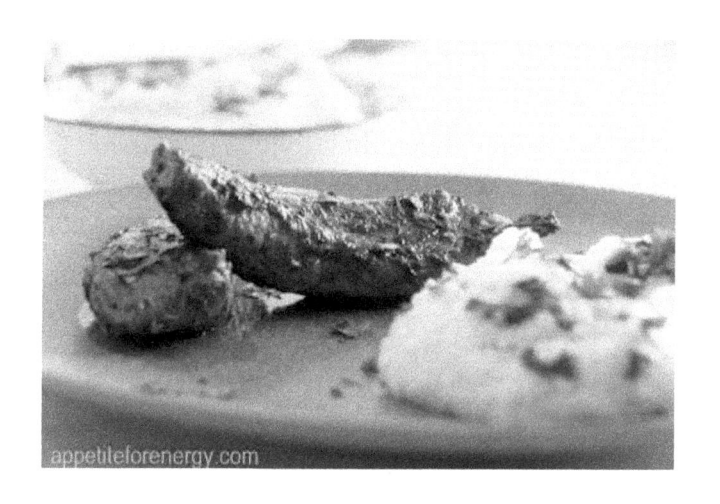

Greek Herbed Lamb is marinated in olive oil, lemon, garlic, oregano and parsley, giving it a fresh, spring taste. Your family will love this tasty, low-carb, 30-minute, Greek lamb recipe!

MACROS PER SERVING:

Calories 714.5, Fat 57.7g, Carbs 16, Protein 34.1g

Prep time: 15 mins
Cook time: 15 mins

Ingredients

Lamb

1. 1.5 lb lamb tenderloin (fillet)
2. 1 tbsp extra virgin olive oil
3. 1 lemon, juiced (2 tbsp)
4. 1/4 tsp pepper
5. 2 tsp dried oregano
6. 1 tsp dried parsley
7. 2-3 crushed garlic cloves
8. Cauliflower Mash
9. 2 lb cauliflower chopped
10. 1 cup light single, pouring cream
11. 3 cups chicken broth
12. 1 oz unsalted butter chopped
13. Himalayan salt

Method

- Make mash: pour cream and chicken stock into a saucepan and turn on the heat. Break the florets off the cauliflower and chop roughly in half, add to the pan.
- Bring to the boil then lower the heat and simmer, covered for 15 mins.
- Once cauliflower is simmering, make the lamb marinade.
- Lamb marinade: Combine all the ingredients except the lamb in a small jug and mix to combine.
- Place lamb in a zip-lock bag and pour over the marinade. Close the bag and jiggle the lamb around so it's well coated. Leave to marinate for about 10 minutes.
- Place a fry-pan over medium-high heat and add 1 tbsp olive oil.

- Pan-fry the lamb for 3-4 minutes on each side. Rest for a few minutes if time permits.

- While the lamb is cooking, drain cauliflower which should be tender by now, reserving 1/4 cup of liquid.

- Use a food processor or immersion blender to blend the cauliflower, butter, salt and the reserved liquid until pureed.

- Serve the Mediterranean lamb with the cauliflower mash.

SEARED TUNA STEAK

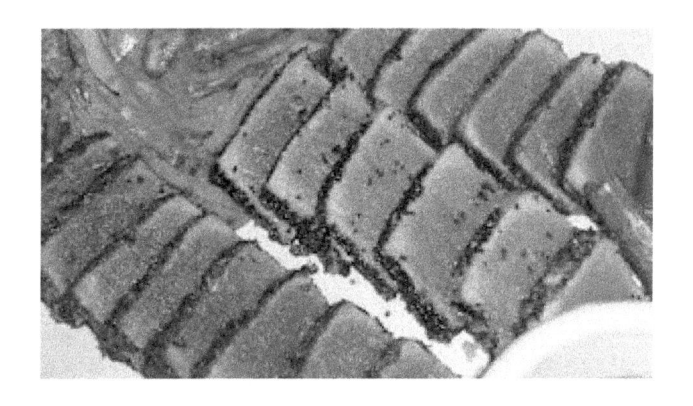

MACROS PER SERVING:

Cals 255, Fat 9g, Protein 40.5g, Carbs 1g

Prep time: 15 minutes
Cook time: 6 minutes

Ingredients

1. 2 (6-ounce) ahi tuna steaks
2. 2 tablespoons soy sauce
3. 1 tablespoon sesame oil
4. 1 teaspoon sesame seeds

5. salt and pepper

Method

- Season the tuna steaks with salt and pepper and place them in a shallow dish.

- Whisk together the soy sauce and sesame oil then pour over the tuna steaks.

- Turn to coat then marinate at room temperature for 15 minutes.

- Heat a large nonstick skillet over medium-high heat until hot.

- Add the tuna steaks and cook for 3 minutes until seared underneath.

- Flip the steaks and cook for another 2 to 3 minutes until done to your liking.

- Slice the steaks in ½-inch slices and garnish with sesame seeds to serve.

QUICK AND EASY RECIPE EASY

BOK CHOY CHICKEN RECIPE

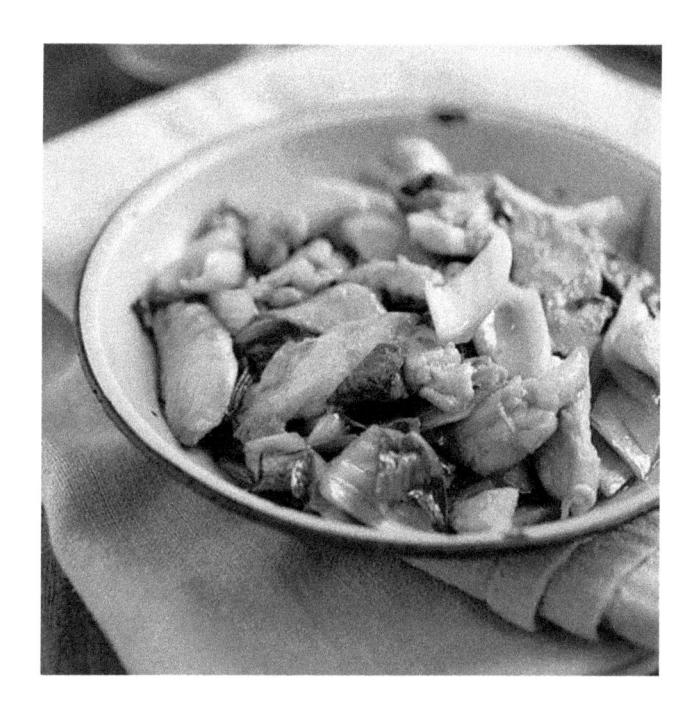

Bok Choy Chicken – easy vegetable stir-fry recipe with bok choy, chicken, garlic and a simple sauce. So EASY, healthy and takes only 15 minutes.

Prep Time 10 minutes

Cook Time 10 minutes
Total Time 20 minutes
Servings 2 people
Calories 188 kcal

Ingredients

1. 6 oz boneless and skinless chicken breast, cut into thin pieces
2. 2 tablespoons oil
3. 8 oz bok choy, sliced into pieces
4. 1 inch piece ginger, peeled and sliced into pieces

Marinade:

5. 1/2 tablespoon soy sauce
6. 1/2 tablespoon cornstarch

Sauce:

7. 1/2 tablespoon oyster sauce
8. 2 tablespoons water

9. 1/4 teaspoon sesame oil

10. 3 dashes white pepper

11. 1 teaspoon wine

12. 1/2 teaspoon sugar

Instructions

- Marinate the chicken with the ingredients in Marinade for 10 minutes. Combine all the ingredients in the Sauce in a small bowl, stir to blend well.

- Heat 1/2 tablespoon oil in a wok until the oil becomes hot. Add the chicken and quickly stir-fry until the surface of the chicken turn opaque or white. Dish out and set aside. This step seals in the juice in the chicken so the texture is tender and vevelty smooth.

- Heat up the remaining oil in the wok until hot. Add the ginger into the wok and stir-fry until aromatic. Add the chicken back into the wok and do a few quick stirs. Add in the bok choy and stir to combine well. Transfer the sauce into the wok and continue to stir-fry until the bok choy is cooked but remain crisp. Do not overcook.

- Dish out and serve immediately with steamed white rice.

Nutrition Facts

- Amount Per Serving (2 people)
- Calories 188
- Fat 144
- Total Fat 16g 25%
- Saturated Fat 1.8g 9%
- Cholesterol 54mg 18%
- Sodium 97mg 4%
- Total Carbohydrates 2.5g 1%
- Dietary Fiber 1.1g 4%
- Sugars 1.3g

- Protein 19.7g 39%

GARLIC BUTTER STEAK RECIPE

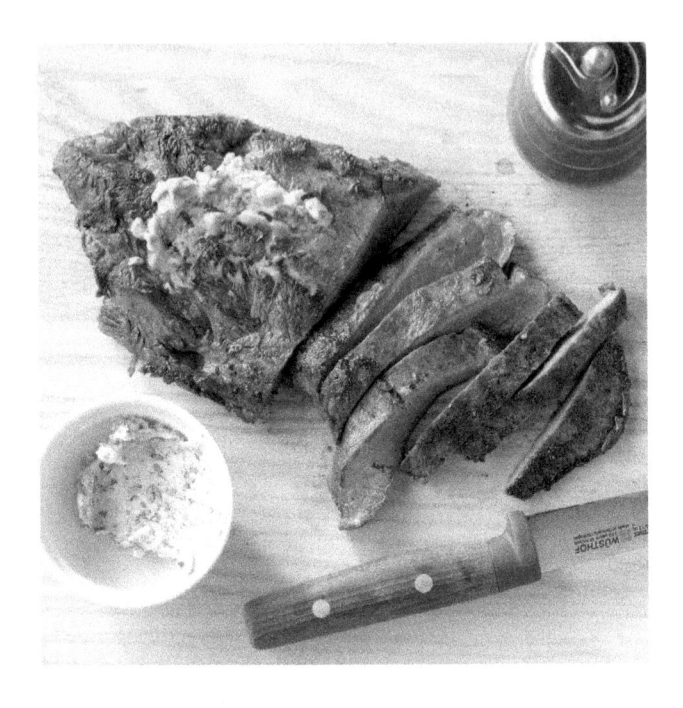

in a cast-iron skillet. Topped with compound garlic butter, this skillet steak recipe is so easy and delicious!

Prep Time 5 minutes
Cook Time 15 minutes
Total Time 20 minutes
Servings 4 people
Calories 248 kcal

Ingredients

1. 12-oz top sirloin steaks (about 1 1/2-inch thick steak)
2. coarse salt
3. ground black pepper
4. 1 tablespoon vegetable oil
5. Garlic Butter
6. 2 tablespoons salted butter, softened
7. 2 cloves garlic, minced
8. 1 tablespoon chopped parsley

Instructions

- Season both sides of the top sirloin steaks generously with salt and ground black pepper. Set aside.

Top Sirloin Steak

- Prepare the Garlic Butter by mixing the butter, garlic and parsley together. Let cool in the fridge.
- Garlic Butter
- Heat up a cast-iron skillet on high heat until smoking hot. Add the oil. Transfer the steak to the skillet and pan-sear each side (do not turn) for about 4 minutes. Turn over and pan-sear the other side for another 4 minutes. Transfer the steak to a serving platter.
- Add a dollop of the Garlic Butter on top of the steak and serve immediately.

Nutrition Facts

Amount Per Serving

- Calories 248
- Total Fat 9g 14%
- Saturated Fat 5g 25%
- Cholesterol 100mg 33%

- Sodium 96mg 4%
- Potassium 607mg 17%
- Protein 38g 76%
- Vitamin A 1.7%
- Vitamin C 2.2%
- Calcium 4%
- Iron 15.6%

PARMESAN GARLIC BREAD RECIPE

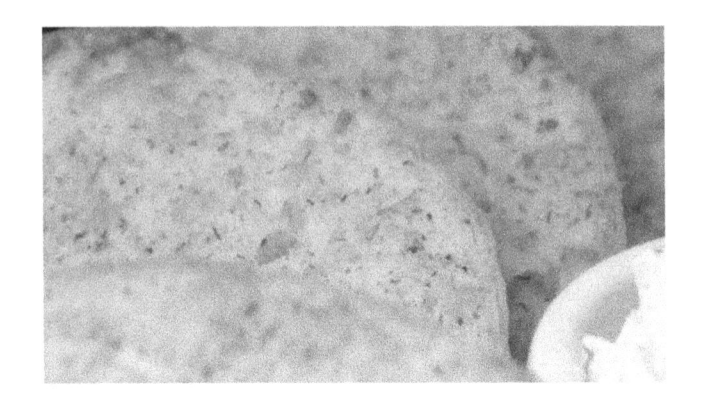

Parmesan Garlic Bread - Turn regular French bread into delicious, buttery parmesan garlic bread with this quick and easy recipe.

Prep Time 10 minutes
Cook Time 15 minutes
Total Time 25 minutes
Servings 3 people
Calories 663 kcal

Ingredients

1. 1 loaf crusty country-style french bread

2. 1 1/4 sticks salted butter, melted

3. 5 cloves garlic, pureed or very finely chopped

4. 5 tablespoons bottled Parmesan cheese

5. 1 teaspoon finely chopped parsley leaves

Instructions

- Preheat the overn to 375F. Slice the horizontally into halves. Set aside.

- In a small bowl, combine the melted butter, garlic, Parmesan cheese and parsley together. Stir to mix well. Brush the mixture generously on the sliced French bread.

- Bake for 15 minutes or until the garlic Parmesan mixture is a bit crusty. Remove from heat, let cool a little bit, and slice into pieces using bread knife. It's best served warm.

Nutrition Facts

- Calories 663
- Total Fat 43g 66%
- Saturated Fat 26g 130%
- Cholesterol 107mg 36%
- Sodium 1155mg 48%
- Potassium 191mg 5%
- Total Carbohydrates 77g 26%
- Dietary Fiber 3g 12%
- Sugars 4g
- Protein 19g 38%
- Vitamin A 24.8%
- Vitamin C 1.9%
- Calcium 17.8%
- Iron 27.7%

GINGER SOY BOK CHOY RECIPE

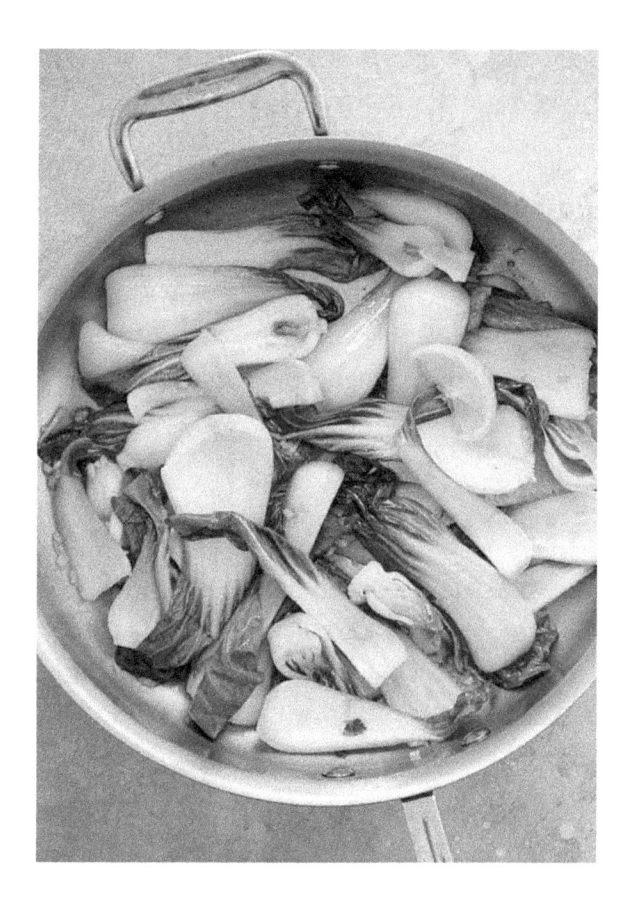

Ginger Soy Bok Choy - the easiest and healthiest bok choy recipe ever. Calls for only 5 ingredients and 10 minutes to make. It's so delicious.

Prep Time 5 minutes
Cook Time 5 minutes
Total Time 10 minutes
Servings 2 people
Calories 94 kcal

Ingredients

1. 1 tablespoons oil
2. 2- inch piece ginger, peeled and minced
3. 12 oz. baby bok choy
4. 1 tablespoon soy sauce
5. 1 teaspoon lemon juice

Instructions

- Rinse the bok choy with cold water, drained. Cut and remove the lower part of the bok choy stems. Cut the (bigger) leaves lengthwise to halves. Set aside.

- Heat up a skillet with the oil. Saute the ginger until aromatic, add the bok choy. Stir fry and toss quickly a few times before adding the soy sauce and lemon juice. As soon as the bok choy are wilted, dish out and serve immediately. DO NOT OVERCOOK.

Nutrition Facts

- Amount Per Serving (2 people)
- Calories 94 Calories from Fat 63
- Total Fat 7g 11%
- Saturated Fat 5g 25%
- Sodium 614mg 26%
- Potassium 48mg 1%
- Total Carbohydrates 5g 2%
- Dietary Fiber 1g 4%
- Sugars 2g
- Protein 2g 4%
- Vitamin A 151.4%
- Vitamin C 94%
- Calcium 18.7% Iron 8%

ASIAN-BRINED PORK CHOPS RECIPE

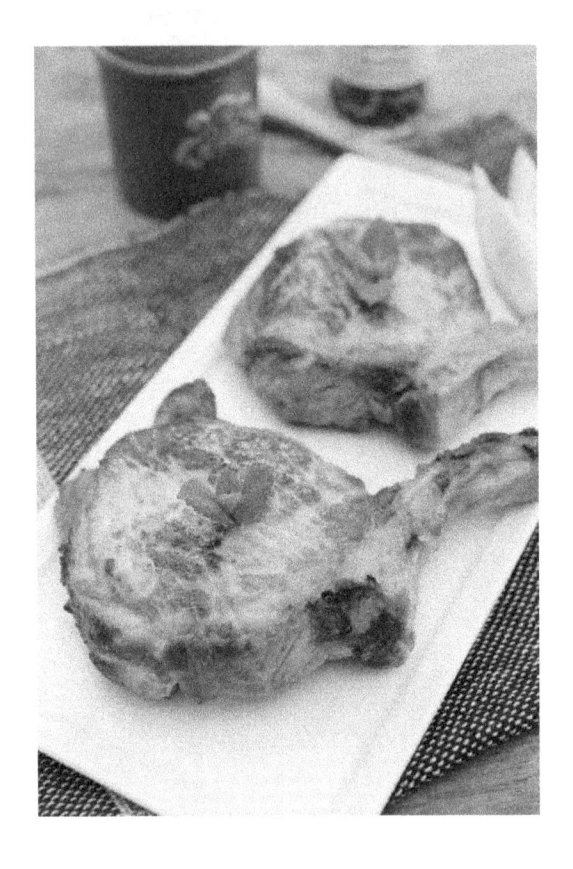

Asian-brined Pork Chops - flavorful and delicious Asian pork chops, so easy to make dinner is ready in 30 mins.

Prep Time 10 minutes
Cook Time 10 minutes
Marinade Time 2 hours
Total Time 20 minutes
Servings 4 people
Calories 482 kcal

Ingredients:

1. 4 bone-in pork chops, 3/4-inch thick
2. 1/8 teaspoon salt or to taste
3. 1 tablespoon cooking oil

Brine:

4. 3/4 cup mirin
5. 1/2 cup low sodium soy sauce
6. 3 ounces fresh ginger, thinly sliced
7. 6-8 small dried chilies
8. 1 orange, thinly sliced
9. 1 1/2 tablespoons sesame oil

10. 1 1/2 cups cold water

11. Garnish (optional):

12. Mint leaves

Instructions

- Lightly season the pork chops with the salt.

- Mix all the ingredients for the Brine in a container or pot, just big enough for the pork chops. Marinade the pork chops in the Brine for at least 2 hours or best overnight.

- Before cooking, remove the pork chops from the Brine and let them come to room temperature. Pat the pork chops dry with paper towels.

- Heat the cooking oil in a non-stick skillet on medium heat. Pan-fry the pork chops for about 4-5 minutes each side. Transfer and wrap the pork chops with foil. Let them rest for 8-10 minutes before serving.

Recipe Notes

- You can choose to use boneless pork chops. Adjust your cooking time accordingly.

Nutrition Facts

- Calories 482
- Total Fat 24g 37%
- Saturated Fat 6g 30%
- Cholesterol 117mg 39%
- Sodium 1575mg 66%
- Potassium 800mg 23%
- Total Carbohydrates 29g 10%
- Dietary Fiber 2g 8%
- Sugars 15g
- Protein 38g 76%
- Vitamin A 5.4%
- Vitamin C 22.7%
- Calcium 5.7%
- Iron 10.5%

GARLIC NOODLES RECIPE

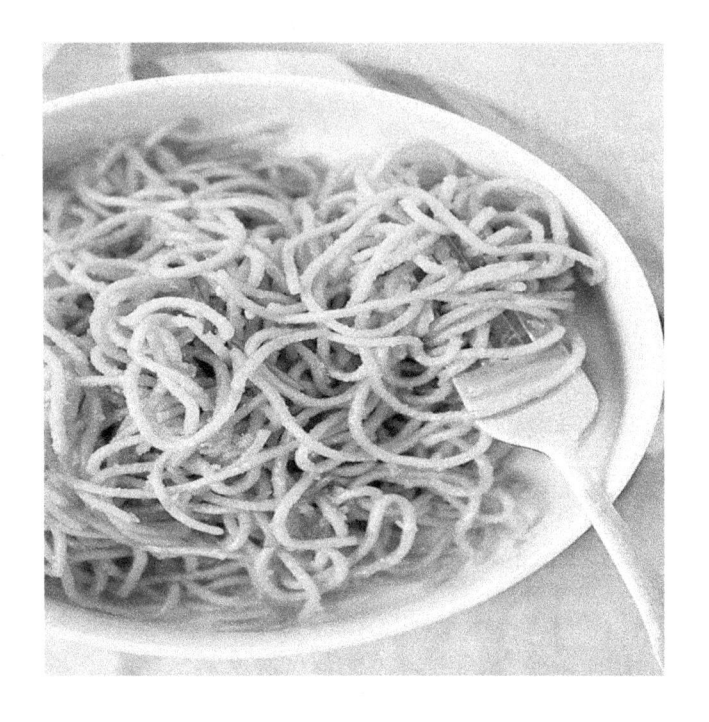

Garlic Noodles - The easiest and best noodles with garlic, butter, Parmesan cheese and Asian seasoning sauces. Tastes just like the best Asian restaurants!

Prep Time 15 minutes
Cook Time 5 minutes
Total Time 20 minutes

Servings 5 people
Calories 604 kcal

Ingredients:

1. 20 oz yellow noodles or spaghetti
2. 1 tablespoon bottled grated Parmesan cheese
3. water, for boiling the noodles

Garlic Sauce:

4. 1 stick unsalted butter (4 oz/110 g/1/2 cup/8 tablespoons)
5. 2 tablespoons minced garlic, or more to taste
6. 1 tablespoon Maggie seasoning sauce
7. 1 tablespoon oyster sauce
8. 1 tablespoon fish sauce
9. 1 tablespoon sugar

Instructions

- Rinse the yellow noodles with running water to discard the oil from the noodles. Drain and set aside.

- Heat up a pot of water until boiling. Add the noodles into the boiling water and cook the noodles until al dente (you want it to still have a good chewy bite), or for a few minutes. You can taste the texture of the noodles while cooking. Do not overcook as the noodles will turn soggy. Transfer the noodles out and drain dry.

- Prepare the garlic sauce using a saute pan on medium to low heat. Add the butter into the pan and when it melts, add the garlic and saute until aromatic but not browned. Add all the seasonings into the pan, stir to combine well. Transfer the garlic sauce into a small bowl.

- To serve, just toss all the noodles with the garlic sauce. Add the cheese, toss to combine well. Serve immediately.

Recipe Notes

- For individual serving of the garlic noodles, take some noodles to a bowl and add some garlic sauce to taste. Drizzle some grated Parmesan cheese, stir to combine well before serving. If you can't find any yellow noodles, you can use spaghetti or linguine.

- Nutrition Facts

- Amount Per Serving (5 people)

- Calories 604

- Total Fat 20g 31%

- Saturated Fat 12g 60%

- Cholesterol 49mg 16%

- Sodium 406mg 17%

- Potassium 276mg 8%

- Total Carbohydrates 88g 29%

- Dietary Fiber 3g 12%

- Sugars 5g
- Protein 15g 30%
- Vitamin A 11.3%
- Vitamin C 1.2%
- Calcium 4.6%
- Iron 8.5%

ROASTED ASPARAGUS WITH GARLIC RECIPE

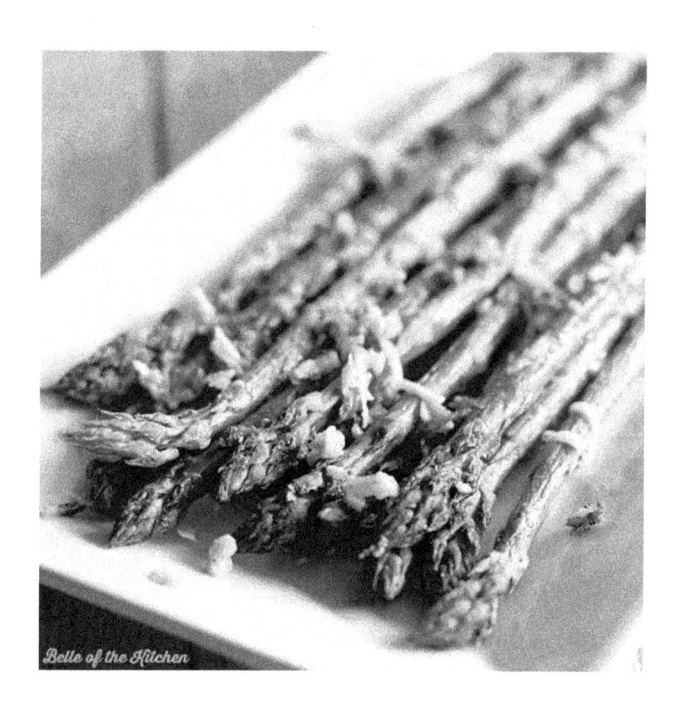

Garlic Roasted Asparagus - healthy oven baked asparagus with garlic. This recipe takes 4 ingredients and only 12 mins to make this quick and easy side dish.

Prep Time 5 minutes
Cook Time 12 minutes

Total Time 17 minutes
Servings 3 people

Ingredients

1. 1 lb asparagus, bottom stems trimmed
2. 2 tablespoons melted salted butter
3. 1 pinch salt
4. 3 cloves garlic, thinly sliced

Instructions

- Preheat oven to 400 F.
- In a sheet pan, toss the asparagus with the melted butter. Season the asparagus with a good pinch of salt. Arrange the garlic slices on top of the asparagus.
- Roast the asparagus for 12 minutes. Remove from oven and serve immediately.

Nutrition Facts

- Amount Per Serving (3 people)
- Calories 98
- Total Fat 7g 11%
- Saturated Fat 4g 20%
- Cholesterol 20mg 7%
- Sodium 70mg 3%
- Potassium 317mg 9%
- Total Carbohydrates 6g 2%
- Dietary Fiber 3g 12%
- Sugars 2g
- Protein 3g 6%
- Vitamin A 27.5%
- Vitamin C 11.4%
- Calcium 4.2%
- Iron 18%

BAKED CHICKEN AND POTATO CASSEROLE RECIPE

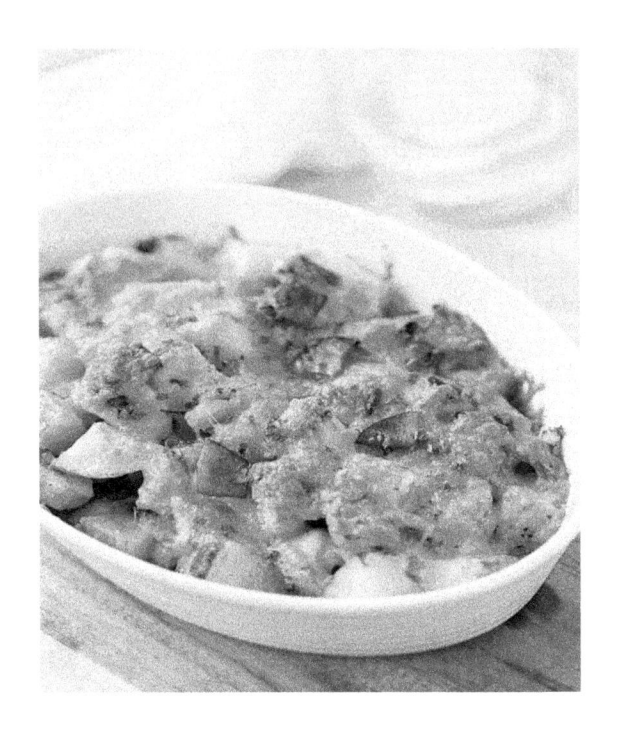

Baked Chicken and Potato Casserole - crazy delicious and easy chicken potato casserole recipe loaded with potatoes, cheddar cheese, bacon and cream.

Prep Time 10 minutes

Cook Time 1 hour 30 minutes
Total Time 1 hour 40 minutes
Servings 2 people
Calories 385 kcal

Ingredients

1. 1/4 teaspoon salt or to taste
2. 1/2 teaspoon sugar
3. 3 dashes ground black pepper
4. 1/4 cup heavy whipping cream
5. 2 medium-sized potatoes, peeled and cut into pieces
6. 8 oz boneless, skinless chicken breasts, cut into cubes
7. 2 slices Canadian bacon, cut into pieces
8. 4 tablespoons unsalted butter, cut into small pieces
9. 1 cup shredded cheddar cheese
10. 1 stalk scallion, green part only, cut into small rounds

Instructions

- Heat oven to 350 degrees F. Lightly grease a 9" x 9" baking pan with some oil or butter.

- Add the salt, sugar, and pepper to the heavy whipping cream. Lightly stir to combine well.

- Spread the potatoes, follow by the chicken, in one single layer. Sprinkle the bacon, butter, and then top with half of the cheddar cheese and the scallions. Pour the heavy cream over top of casserole. Cover with aluminum foil and bake for 1 hour. Uncover the pan and bake for another 30 minutes. In the last 10 minutes, sprinkle with the remaining cheddar cheese and bake until the cheese is slightly crusty. Remove from the oven and serve immediately.

Recipe Notes

- Instead of Canadian bacon, you can use 1 or 2 strips of bacon. If you use bacon, pre-cooked them until they are crisp first.

- Nutrition Facts
- Amount Per Serving (2 people)
- Calories 385
- Total Fat 64g 98%
- Saturated Fat 37g 185%
- Cholesterol 247mg 82%
- Sodium 956mg 40%
- Potassium 1440mg 41%
- Total Carbohydrates 31g 10%
- Dietary Fiber 6g 24%
- Sugars 1g
- Protein 48g 96%
- Vitamin A 35.9%
- Vitamin C 32.4%
- Calcium 51%
- Iron 43.6%

ITALIAN SHRIMP PASTA RECIPE

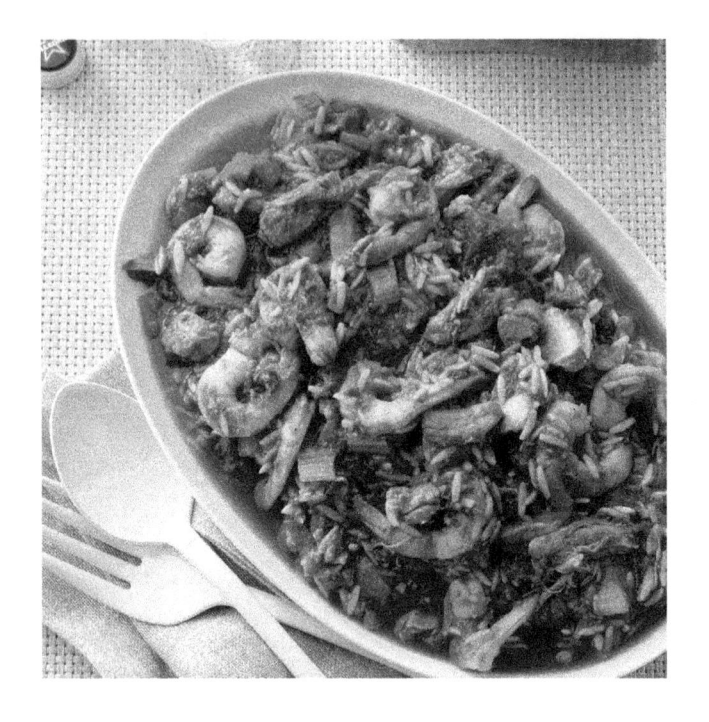

This is a proper Italian Shrimp Pasta recipe, the authentic way Italian home cooks and chefs make shrimp pasta. The pasta is fresh, healthy, with an absolutely mouthwatering homemade tomato sauce.

Prep Time 10 minutes

Cook Time 10 minutes
Total Time 20 minutes
Servings 2 people
Calories 392 kcal

Ingredients

1. 4 oz spaghetti pasta
2. 2 tablespoons extra virgin olive oil
3. 3 cloves garlic, finely minced
4. 4 oz Campari tomatoes, cut into thin wedges
5. 1/4 cup chicken broth
6. 1/2 teaspoon chicken bouillon
7. 4 oz peeled and deveined shrimp or jumbo prawn, butterflied
8. 3/4 teaspoon salt or more to taste
9. freshly ground black pepper
10. 1 teaspoon chopped Italian parsley

Instructions

- Bring a pot of salted water to boil. Cook the spaghetti al dente, according to package instruction.

- In a skillet or pan on medium-low heat, add the extra virgin olive oil. Saute the garlic until sizzling but not browned. Add the tomatoes, chicken broth and chicken bouillon. As soon as it bubbles, add the shrimp. Cook and stir until the shrimps are cooked and the tomatoes break down.

- Add the spaghetti, salt and generous dose of freshly ground black pepper. Stir to combine well. Turn off the heat.

- Top the Shrimp Pasta with chopped Italian parsley and serve immediately.

Nutrition Facts

- Amount Per Serving (2 people)
- Calories 392

- Total Fat 15g 23%
- Saturated Fat 2g 10%
- Cholesterol 71mg 24%
- Sodium 1312mg 55%
- Potassium 366mg 10%
- Total Carbohydrates 46g 15%
- Dietary Fiber 2g 8%
- Sugars 3g
- Protein 16g 32%
- Vitamin A 11.5%
- Vitamin C 13.6%
- Calcium 5.6%
- Iron 5.6%

GARLIC PARMESAN ROASTED CARROTS RECIPE

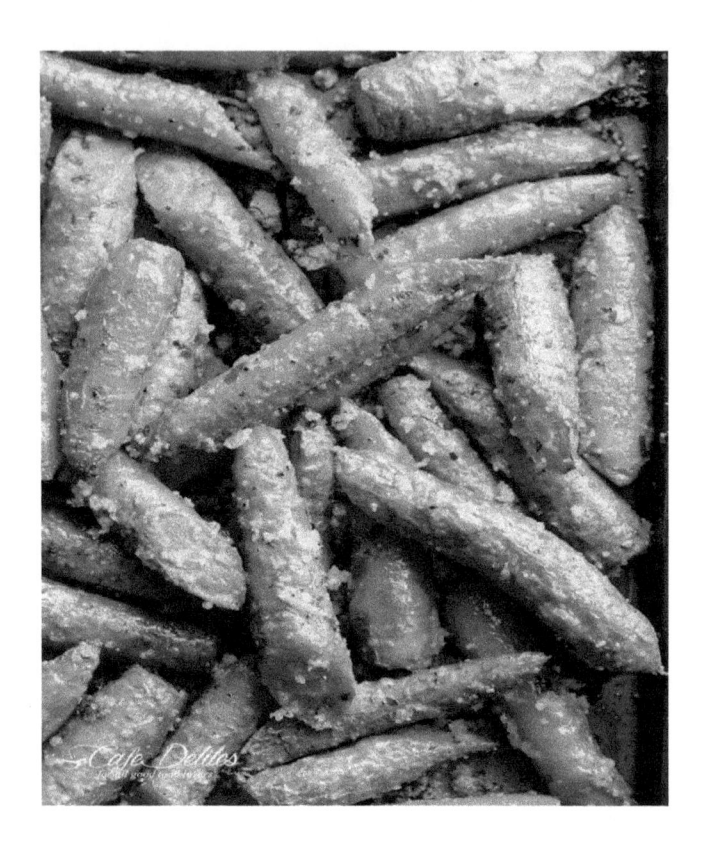

Garlic Parmesan Roasted Carrots - oven roasted carrots with butter, garlic and Parmesan cheese. The easiest and most delicious carrot recipes ever!

Prep Time 10 minutes
Cook Time 25 minutes
Total Time 35 minutes
Servings 2 people
Calories 186 kcal

Ingredients

1. 12 oz carrots, skin peeled
2. 2 tablespoons melted salted butter
3. 2 cloves garlic, minced
4. 3 tablespoons grated Parmesan cheese
5. 1 teaspoon chopped parsley

Instructions

- Preheat the oven to 400F.
- Mix the melted butter and garlic together. Coat the carrots well with the butter mixture.
- Arrange the carrots on a baking sheet lined with parchment paper. Drizzle the extra

butter garlic mixture on top of the carrots. Roast for 15 minutes, then top the carrots with the Parmesan cheese. Roast for another 10 minutes or until the cheese melts and slightly browned. Remove from the oven and top with the parsley. Serve immediately.

Recipe Notes

- For sweet versions of carrots, please try my honey butter roasted carrots, maple butter roasted baby carrots or candied carrots.

Nutrition Facts

- Amount Per Serving (2 people)
- Calories 186
- Total Fat 14g 22%
- Saturated Fat 9g 45%
- Cholesterol 37mg 12%
- Sodium 333mg 14%

- Potassium 544mg 16%
- Total Carbohydrates 18g 6%
- Dietary Fiber 5g 20%
- Sugars 8g
- Protein 5g 10%
- Vitamin A 576.6%
- Vitamin C 13.3%
- Calcium 14.5%
- Iron 2.8%

GARLIC HERB GRILLED SALMON RECIPE

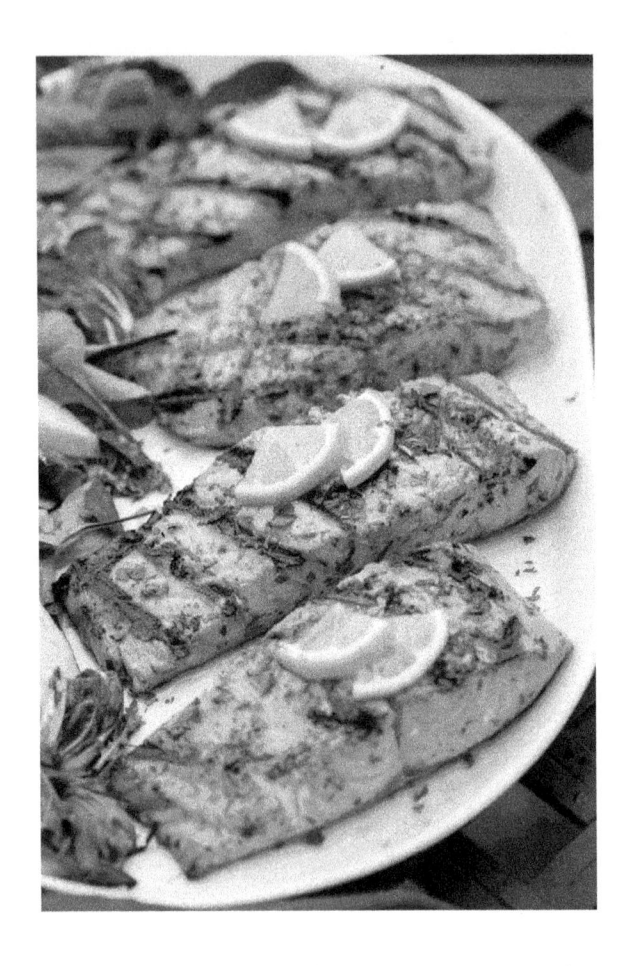

Garlic Herb Grilled Salmon - moist and juicy salmon with garlic, herbs, olive oil and lemon marinade. This is the best grilled salmon recipe ever and takes only 8 minutes on gas grill.

Prep Time 10 minutes
Cook Time 8 minutes
Marinade Time 20 minutes
Total Time 38 minutes
Servings 4 people
Calories 228 kcal

Ingredients

1. 1 lb. salmon (top loin, loin or second cut)
2. lemon wedges, for serving
3. Marinade:
4. 2 tablespoons olive oil
5. 2 cloves garlic, minced
6. 1 teaspoon chopped Italian basil
7. 1 tablespoon chopped Italian parsley
8. 1 tablespoon lemon juice
9. 1/2 teaspoon salt

10. 3 dashes ground black pepper

Instructions

- Mix all the Marinade ingredients in a bowl, stir to mix well.

- Marinate the salmon with the Marinade for 20 minutes.

- Salmon fillet in grilled salmon marinade.

- Heat up a gas grill to medium heat, at 350 degrees F. Remove the marinated salmon from the Marinade and place it on top of the gas grill. Place the salmon, skin side down at a 45 degree angle to form beautiful char marks. Grill the salmon for 4 minutes, uninterrupted. Turn the salmon over and grill for another 4 minutes, uninterrupted. Baste with the remaining Marinade mixture while grilling.

- Grilling salmon with skin on a gas grill.

- Depending on the type of salmon cuts you use, you might need to grill it for longer (or shorter) time. The salmon is cooked when white stuff starts to seep out from the inside. If the salmon is not cooked yet but already charred, move the salmon to the indirect heat side of the gas grill. Cover the lid and cook for 1-2 minutes or until the inside is completely cooked through. Remove from the grill and serve immediately with lemon wedges, dill sauce, or sweet chili sauce.

Nutrition Facts

- Amount Per Serving (4 people)
- Calories 228
- Total Fat 14g 22%
- Saturated Fat 2g 10%
- Cholesterol 62mg 21%
- Sodium 342mg 14%

- Potassium 566mg 16%
- Total Carbohydrates 1g 0%
- Dietary Fiber 1g 4%
- Sugars 1g
- Protein 23g 46%
- Vitamin A 2.6%
- Vitamin C 3.9%
- Calcium 2%
- Iron 5.8%

BAKED CHICKEN WINGS RECIPE

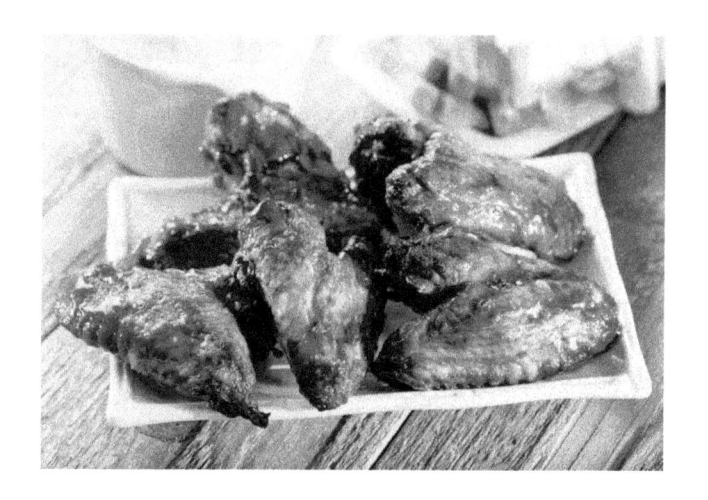

Delicious honey baked chicken wings with 5 ingredients and 5 minutes active time. This is an easy chicken wings recipe in oven that anyone can make at home.

Prep Time 5 minutes
Cook Time 30 minutes
Total Time 35 minutes
Servings 3 people
Calories 325 kcal

Ingredients

1. 1/2 lbs chicken wings (drummettes and wingettes)
2. 2 tablespoons A1 Steak Sauce, Original
3. 2 tablespoons honey
4. 1/2 teaspoon salt
5. 3 dashes cayenne pepper

Instructions

- Preheat oven to 400 degrees F.
- In the meantime, add the A1 sauce, honey, salt and cayenne pepper to the chicken wings. Stir to mix well.
- Transfer the chicken to a baking sheet lined with parchment paper, arrange in single layer. Spoon the remaining marinade sauce on each chicken wing.
- Bake the chicken wings in the oven for 30 minutes, or until the surface turns crispy and brown. Remove from oven and serve immediately with your favorite dipping sauce.

Nutrition Facts

- Amount Per Serving (3 people)
- Calories 325
- Total Fat 20g 31%
- Saturated Fat 6g 30%
- Cholesterol 94mg 31%
- Sodium 643mg 27%
- Potassium 242mg 7%
- Total Carbohydrates 14g 5%
- Dietary Fiber 1g 4%
- Sugars 13g
- Protein 23g 46%
- Vitamin A 12.5%
- Vitamin C 2.8%
- Calcium 1.5%
- Iron 7.7%

SWEET AND SOUR PORK NOODLES RECIPE

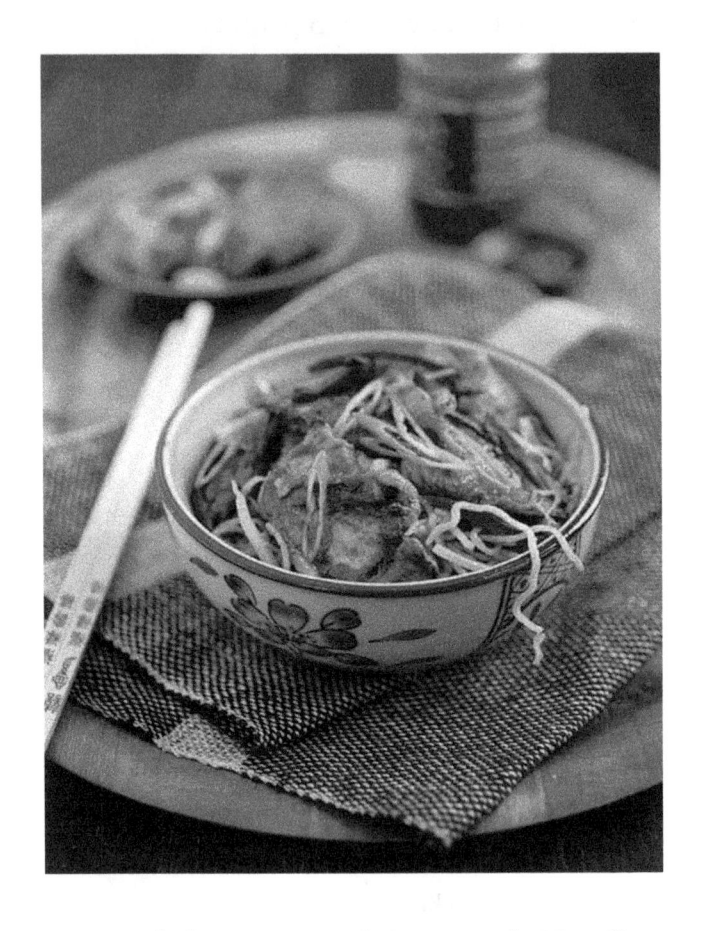

Super Delish Sweet and Sour Pork Noodles – sweet and sour flavor, with pork and noodles. Your tummy will be happy with this tried and tested recipe.

Prep Time 10 minutes
Cook Time 10 minutes
Total Time 20 minutes
Servings 2 people
Calories 656 kcal

Ingredients:

1. 8 oz egg noodles
2. 4 oz pork, sliced into thin pieces
3. 2 tablespoons oil
4. 2 cloves garlic, minced
5. 4 oz bean sprouts, roots removed (optional)
6. 1/2 tablespoon oyster sauce
7. Salt to taste
8. Marinade:
9. 1/2 tablespoon soy sauce

10. 1/4 teaspoon sesame oil

11. 3 dashes white pepper

12. 1 teaspoon garlic chili sauce

13. 1/2 tablespoon sugar

14. 1 teaspoon vinegar

Instructions

- Boil the egg noodles until al dente. Rinse quickly with cold water, drained dry and set aside.

- Marinate the pork with all the ingredients in the Marinade, for 15 minutes.

- Heat up the oil in a wok or skillet. When the oil is heated, add the garlic and stir fry until aromatic. Add the pork into the wok, stir and cook until they are almost cooked. Add the bean sprouts, follow by the noodles. Add the oyster sauce. Stir to combine well with noodles and all the ingredients in the work or skillet, add a little salt to taste. When the bean sprouts are wilted and cooked but remain crunchy, the dish is ready to be served.

Nutrition Facts

- Calories 656
- Total Fat 32g 49%
- Saturated Fat 17g 85%
- Cholesterol 136mg 45%
- Sodium 557mg 23%
- Potassium 524mg 15%
- Total Carbohydrates 91g 30%
- Dietary Fiber 5g 20%
- Sugars 8g
- Protein 28g 56%
- Vitamin A 1.4%
- Vitamin C 10.2%
- Calcium 6%
- Iron 19.4%

CRISPY BAKED ORANGE CHICKEN WINGS RECIPE

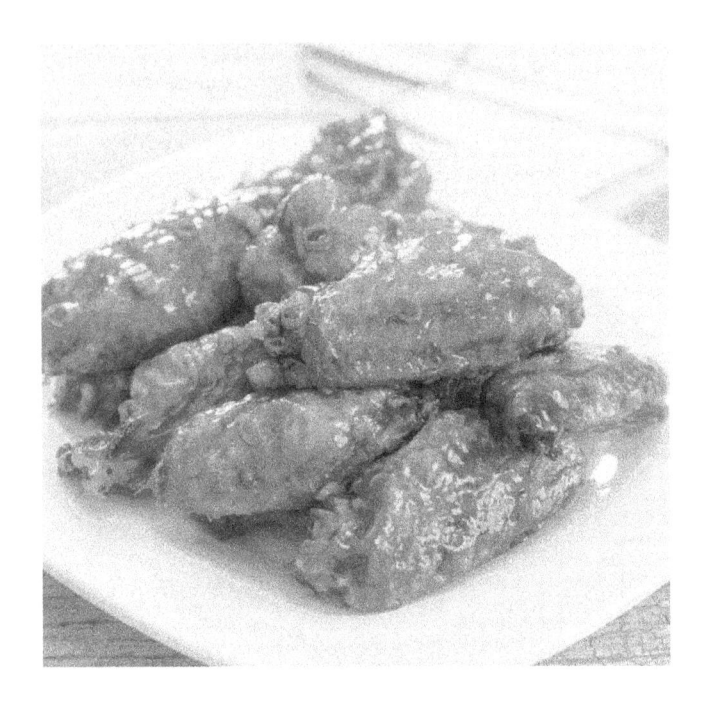

Baked Orange Chicken Wings - crispy, sticky baked wings (no frying) in an amazeballs orange sauce, so yummy.

Prep Time 15 minutes
Cook Time 50 minutes
Total Time 1 hour 5 minutes

Servings 4 people
Calories 342 kcal

Ingredients

1. 2 lbs chicken wings, tips removed, drumettes and middle sections separated
2. 1 tablespoon oil
3. Salt
4. Black Pepper
5. Orange Sauce:
6. 1/4 cup orange juice
7. 1/2 teaspoon orange zest
8. 1 tablespoon Rooster brand Huy Fong Garlic Chili Sauce, (optional)
9. 3 tablespoons chicken broth or water
10. 1 tablespoon soy sauce
11. 5 teaspoons sugar

12. 1 teaspoon Apple cider vinegar, red wine or Chinese white vinegar

13. 2 teaspoons Chinese rice wine or dry sherry, (optional)

14. 1 teaspoon cornstarch

<u>Instructions</u>

- Preheat oven to 400ºF.

- Rinse the chicken wings and pat dry with paper towels. Transfer to a large bowl and toss with the oil, some salt and black pepper. Line a baking tray with aluminum foil and then place a baking rack on top. Arrange the wings in a single layer on the rack, as pictured below.

- Bake, rotating pan half-way through, until fully cooked and crispy, about 45 to 50 minutes. Make sure you keep checking on them.

- Mix all the ingredients in the Orange Sauce in sauce pan. Heat it up until it thickens and slightly bubbles. Turn off the heat and set aside.

- When the chicken are done, transfer them out of the oven and add to the Orange Sauce. Toss a few times to coat well.

- Drizzle some sesame seeds and chopped cilantro on top of the chicken wings. Serve immediately.

Nutrition Facts

- Amount Per Serving (4 people)
- Calories 342
- Total Fat 23g 35%
- Saturated Fat 8g 40%
- Cholesterol 94mg 31%
- Sodium 591mg 25%
- Potassium 240mg 7%
- Total Carbohydrates 8g 3%

- Sugars 7g
- Protein 23g 46%
- Vitamin A 4.2%
- Vitamin C 11.8%
- Calcium 1.5%
- Iron 7.1%

POMELO SALAD: YAM SOM-O RECIPE

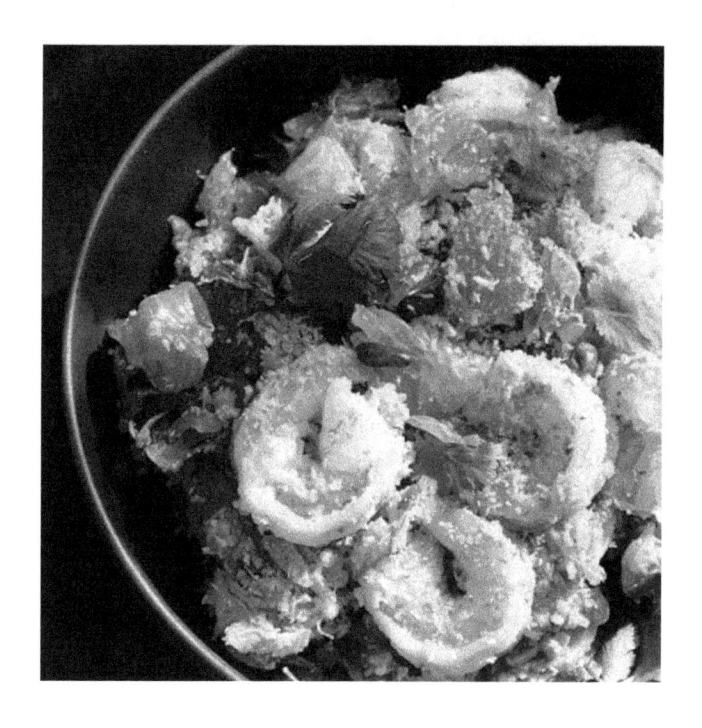

Thai Pomelo Salad recipe (Yam Som-O) - coconut flakes, shrimp, red chili flakes, shallots, garlic, roasted peanuts, lime juice, cilantro.

Servings 4 people
Calories 420 kcal

Ingredients

1. 1.5 lb pomelo, peeled and separated into segments
2. 1 lb 21-26 count shrimp, peeled and deveined
3. ¾ cup desiccated coconut flakes, unsweetened
4. ½ cup coconut milk
5. Dried red chile flakes, to taste (I use whole Mexican chile pequin as they are very easy to crumble up with your fingertips and taste just like dried bird's eye chiles. They're also very, very cute.)
6. 4 tablespoons finely-minced shallots or onion
7. 2 tablespoons finely-minced garlic
8. 2 tablespoons vegetable oil
9. ½ cup plain roasted peanuts, roughly chopped
10. fresh lime juice to taste
11. fish sauce, to taste

12. 1 handful fresh cilantro leaves fish sauce

Instructions

- In a small saucepan, sauté together the vegetable oil, shallots, garlic, and dried pepper flakes over medium heat until the mixture releases its wonderful aroma and becomes confit-like in consistency. Add the coconut milk into the shallot mixture and heat through; remove from heat and set aside to cool.

- In a skillet over medium-low heat, dry toast the desiccated coconut flakes until they turn medium brown color. Be careful not to leave the skillet unattended; coconut burns very easily. Set the toasted coconut aside to cool.

- Poach the shrimp, drain, and set it aside.

- Gently break up the pomelo segments into roughly ½-inch pieces and put them in a large mixing bowl.

- Add the poached shrimp, shallot-coconut mixture, toasted coconut flakes, peanuts, and cilantro leaves to the pomelo bowl.

- Add to the mixing bowl 2 tablespoons each of the lime juice and fish sauce and toss everything together as gently as you can with your hands . Adjust the seasoning with more lime juice or fish sauce as needed. (If your pomelo is on the tart side, you may want to add just a tiny bit of sugar to counteract the acidity. But usually the subtle, natural sweetness of the toasted coconut and coconut milk is sufficient.)

- Serve immediately with additional roasted peanuts and toasted coconut on top, if desired.

- Recipe Notes

- Though quite a few recipe authors suggest grapefruit as a substitute for pomelo, I encourage you to seek out pomelo in Hispanic or Asian stores in your area first. Then, if you absolutely cannot find it, use grapefruit segments, blotted dry with a clean kitchen towel to remove as much juice as possible. (Grapefruit releases a lot of juice and I don't like a salad that swims in juices.) Navel orange segments can also be used. (But then you can't really call it Yam Som-O since the Som-O is absent.

- Make sure that the roasted peanuts are fresh. Nothing ruins an otherwise good dish like rancid peanuts.

- The best way to poach shrimp is in simmering, not furiously boiling, water at the temperature of 160° and 180°F (71–82°C). Be sure to not overcook the shrimp.

- Do not substitute lemon juice for lime juice, soy sauce for fish sauce, or sweet coconut flakes for plain desiccated coconut.

- To kick it up a notch, add to the mix 2-3 tablespoons of crispy-fried shallots, commercial or homemade.

Nutrition Facts

- Amount Per Serving (4 people)
- Calories 420
- Total Fat 33g 51%
- Saturated Fat 21g 105%
- Cholesterol 142mg 47%
- Sodium 732mg 31%
- Potassium 467mg 13%
- Total Carbohydrates 11g 4%
- Dietary Fiber 4g 16%
- Sugars 2g
- Protein 22g 44%
- Vitamin A 4.1%
- Vitamin C 3.1%
- Calcium 10%
- Iron 12.8%

ONE POT MEATBALL CASSEROLE RECIPE

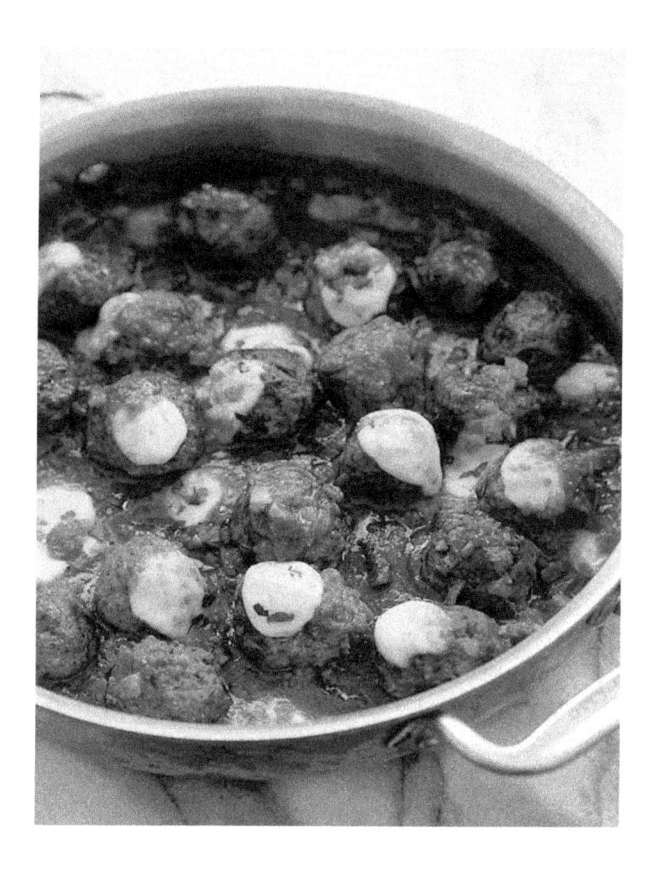

Meatball Casserole – one pot juicy and delicious meatballs in tomato sauce and topped with mozzarella cheese, homemade comfort food.

Prep Time 40 minutes
Cook Time 10 minutes
Total Time 50 minutes
Servings 4
Calories 713 kcal

Ingredients

1. 1 lb. ground pork
2. 1 lb. ground beef
3. 1 cup breadcrumbs or Japanese panko
4. 1/2 cup finely grated Parmesan cheese
5. 1 1/2 teaspoons Kosher salt
6. 2 large eggs
7. 1 clove garlic minced
8. 1/4 cup chopped flat-leaf parsley
9. 2 tablespoons extra-virgin olive oil
10. 1/2 small onion finely chopped
11. Pinch of red-pepper flakes
12. 1 can 28 oz. whole peeled tomatoes, pureed

13. 4 fresh basil leaves optional

14. 8 oz fresh mozzarella cheese thinly sliced

Instructions

- Using your hands, gently mix together the pork, beef, breadcrumbs, Parmesan cheese, salt, eggs, garlic, and parsley in a large bowl. Form mixture into 2-inch balls.

- Heat the oil in a large oven-safe skillet over medium-high heat. Add the meatballs; cook, turning, until browned all over, about 10 minutes. Use a slotted spoon to transfer to a plate.

- Reduce the heat to medium. Add onion and pepper flakes; cook, stirring occasionally, until onion is tender. Add the tomatoes and basil; simmer, stirring frequently, until the sauce is slightly thickened. Return the meatballs and its juices to pan. Simmer, turning meatballs until cooked through.

- Heat the broiler and arrange the mozzarella cheese on top of the meatballs. Broil until melted, about 2 minutes. Serve immediately.

Nutrition Facts

- Amount Per Serving (4 g)
- Calories 713
- Total Fat 337g 518%
- Saturated Fat 14.1g 71%
- Cholesterol 275mg 92%
- Sodium 1746mg 73%
- Total Carbohydrates 23.7g 8%
- Dietary Fiber 1.6g 6%
- Sugars 2.3g
- Protein 77.4g 155%

THAI PEANUT ZUCCHINI NOODLES RECIPE

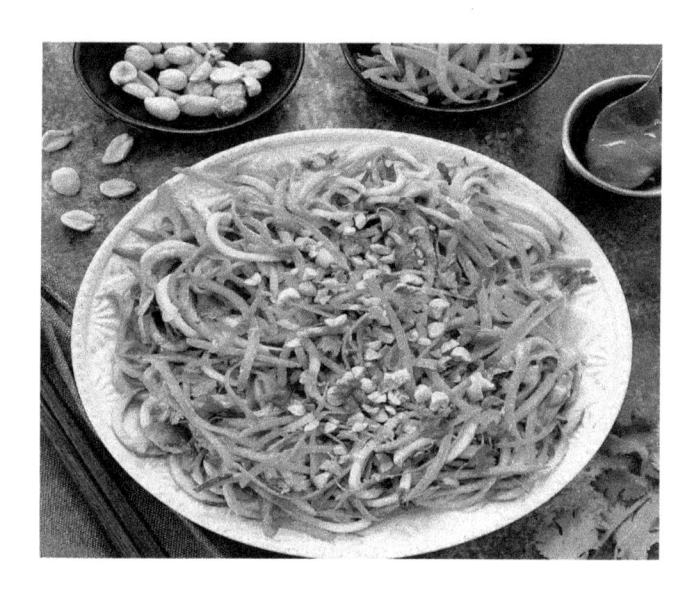

Thai Peanut Zucchini Noodles - easy and healthy recipe with veggie noodles in mouthwatering Thai peanut sauce. This recipe is delicious and takes 15 mins to make.

Prep Time 20 minutes
Total Time 20 minutes
Servings 3 people
Calories 305 kcal

Ingredients

1. 1 lb. zucchini
2. 4 oz. carrots, peeled
3. 2 oz. spaghetti, (optional)
4. 4 tablespoons creamy peanut butter
5. 4 tablespoons Thai sweet chili sauce
6. 2 tablespoons apple cider vinegar
7. 1 tablespoon chopped peanuts

Instructions

- Trim both ends of the zucchini and attach it to a spiralizer and make the zucchini into noodles. Attach the carrots to the spiralizer and make the carrot noodles. Discard any water that seeps out from the the veggie noodles.

- Cook the spaghetti according to package instructions, if using. Drain and set aside. Mix all noodles together.

- Make the Thai peanut sauce by mixing the peanut butter, sweet chili sauce, vinegar together into a runny dressing.
- Toss the veggie noodles with the peanut sauce gently. Don't over mix. Top the noodles with crushed peanuts and serve immediately.

Recipe Notes

- The spaghetti is optional, but I used it in my recipe above. Spaghetti makes it a more substantial meal but you can opted out if you want a lighter meal.

Nutrition Facts

- Amount Per Serving (3 people)
- Calories 305
- Total Fat 13g 20%
- Saturated Fat 2g 10%
- Sodium 387mg 16%

- Potassium 718mg 21%
- Total Carbohydrates 38g 13%
- Dietary Fiber 4g 16%
- Sugars 19g
- Protein 10g 20%
- Vitamin A 132.3%
- Vitamin C 35.5%
- Calcium 5%
- Iron 7.7%

TANDOORI CHICKEN RECIPE

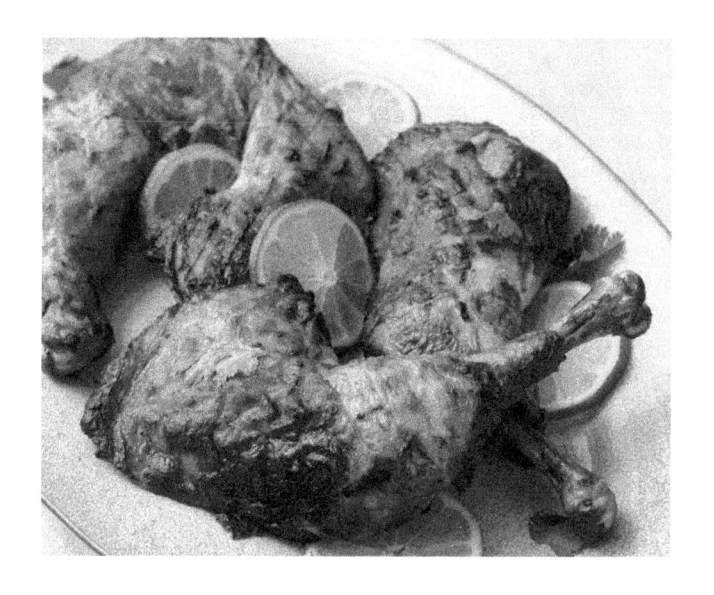

The best homemade oven-baked tandoori chicken recipe ever! This authentic Tandoori chicken is tender, moist, juicy and a zillion times better than Indian buffets!

Prep Time 15 minutes
Cook Time 40 minutes
Marinade Time 2 hours
Servings 3 people
Calories 259 kcal

Ingredients

1. 1 lb chicken legs
2. Oil, for basting
3. 1 lime, cut into wedges

Marinade:

4. 1/2 cup Greek yogurt
5. 1 teaspoon ginger, finely minced
6. 1 teaspoon garlic, finely minced
7. 1/2 teaspoon Garam Masala
8. 1/4 teaspoon cayenne pepper
9. 2 tablespoons lime juice
10. 1 tablespoons oil
11. 1 1/2 teaspoons salt or to taste, (optional)
12. 1/4 teaspoon turmeric powder
13. Red coloring, (optional)

Instructions

- Clean and pat dry the chicken with paper towels.

- Mix all the ingredients of the Marinade in a bowl. Stir to combine well. Add the chicken to the Marinade and marinate for at least 2 hours, or best 4 hours.

- Preheat the oven to 400°F. Line the baking sheet with aluminum foil and place a wire rack over it. Place the chicken on the wire rack. Bake for 20 minutes, then turn the chicken over and bake for another 20 minutes. Using a small brush, baste both surfaces of the chicken with the oil a couple of times during baking. Broil the chicken for 1 minute or until the skin is slightly charred. Remove from the oven and serve immediately with lime wedges.

Recipe Notes

- Serve the Tandoori chicken with Naan

Nutrition Facts

- Tandoori Chicken Recipe
- Amount Per Serving (3 people)
- Calories 259
- Total Fat 18g 28%
- Saturated Fat 4g 20%
- Cholesterol 81mg 27%
- Sodium 1248mg 52%
- Potassium 244mg 7%
- Total Carbohydrates 5g 2%
- Sugars 1g
- Protein 17g 34%
- Vitamin A 3%
- Vitamin C 11.9%
- Calcium 5.2%
- Iron 4.4%

SPAM FRIED RICE RECIPE

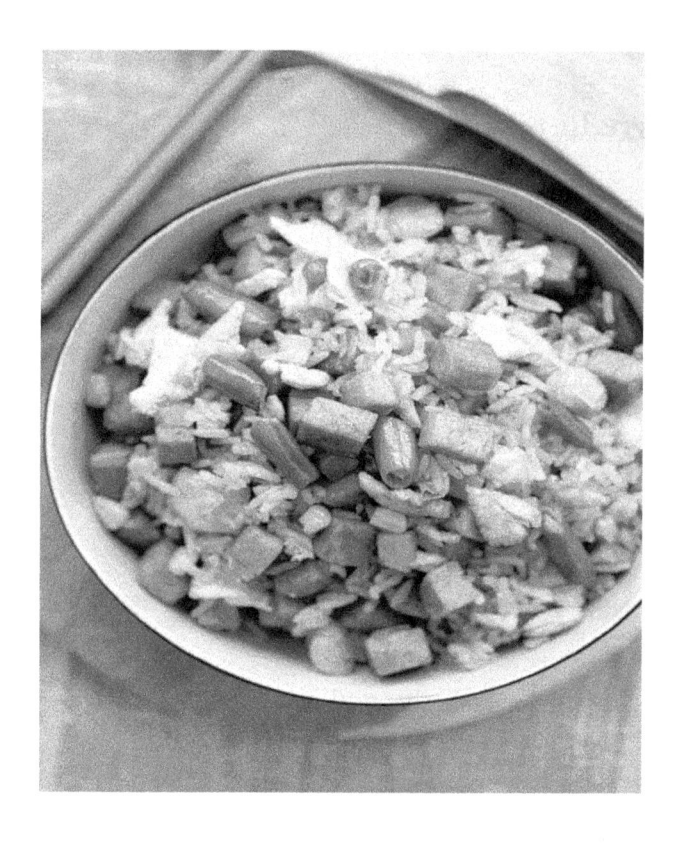

Fried rice with spam, eggs and mixed vegetables in this quick and easy Spam fried rice recipe that you can make at home in a jiffy. This is the best!

Prep Time 10 minutes
Cook Time 10 minutes

Total Time 20 minutes
Servings 4 people
Calories 481 kcal

Ingredients

1. 3 cups overnight steamed rice
2. 2 1/2 tablespoons oil
3. 3 large eggs, lightly beaten
4. 2 cloves garlic, minced
5. 6 oz spam, cut into small cubes
6. 1 cup frozen mixed vegetables, thaw and defrost
7. salt, to taste

Seasonings:

8. 1 1/2 tablespoons soy sauce
9. 1/2 tablespoon fish sauce
10. 1/2 teaspoon sesame oil
11. 3 dashes ground white pepper

Instructions

- Break up the lumpy overnight rice with the back of the spoon or fork, or with your hand. Mix all the ingredients for the Seasonings in a small bowl.

- Heat 1/2 tablespoon of the oil in a wok over high heat and cook the eggs first. Use the spatula to break the eggs into small pieces. Set aside. Reheat the wok with the remaining 2 tablespoons oil and stir-fry the garlic until aromatic. Add the spam pieces and stir-fry until light brown before adding the mixed vegetables. Stir to combine well.

- Add the rice into the wok and use the spatula to stir-fry continuously until the all the ingredients are well blended. Add the Seasonings into the wok, blending it well with the rice and ingredients. Return the cooked eggs into the wok and combine with the rice. Dish out and serve immediately.

Nutrition Facts

- Spam Fried Rice Recipe
- Amount Per Serving (4 people)
- Calories 481
- Total Fat 24g 37%
- Saturated Fat 13g 65%
- Cholesterol 153mg 51%
- Sodium 1222mg 51%
- Potassium 367mg 10%
- Total Carbohydrates 50g 17%
- Dietary Fiber 2g 8%
- Sugars 1g
- Protein 16g 32%
- Vitamin A 49.8%
- Vitamin C 6.3%
- Calcium 3.3%
- Iron 19.9%

KUNG PAO SHRIMP RECIPE

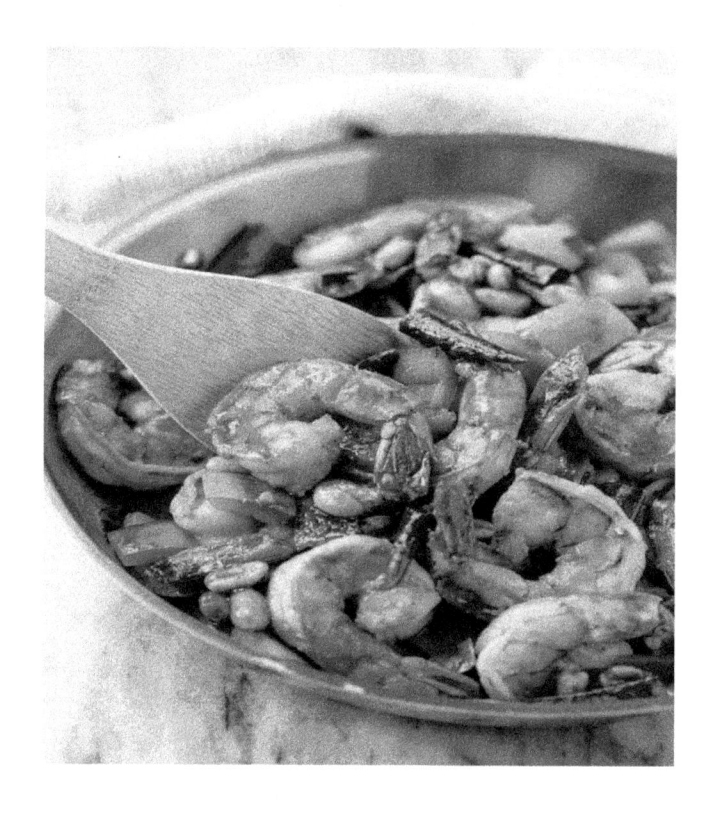

Kung Pao Shrimp - easy and delicious Kung Pao shrimp recipe that takes 20 mins to make. This recipe is so much better and healthier than Chinese takeout.

Prep Time 15 minutes

Cook Time 5 minutes
Total Time 20 minutes
Servings 2 people
Calories 457 kcal

Ingredients

1. 2 tablespoons oil
2. 1 inch piece ginger, peeled and thinly sliced
3. 1/4 onion, quartered
4. 1/2 green bell pepper, cut into pieces
5. 10 mini dried red chilies, (5 regular-sized dried chilies)
6. 10-12 oz big shrimp, shelled, peeled and deveined
7. 1/4 cup roasted peanuts
8. 3 stalks scallions, use the white parts only
9. Kung Pao Sauce:
10. 2 tablespoons soy sauce
11. 2 tablespoons sweet soy sauce, (ABC Kecap Manis)

12. 1/2 teaspoon corn starch

13. 4 tablespoons water

14. 1/2 teaspoon sesame oil

15. 3 dashes white pepper

16. 1/2 teaspoon Chinese black vinegar, rice vinegar or apple cider vinegar

17. 1/2 teaspoon sugar

Instructions

- Mix the Kung Pao sauce ingredients and set aside.

- Heat up a wok and add the cooking oil until the oil is very hot. Add the ginger and do a few quick stirs. Add the onion, green pepper, and dried red chilies. Stir-fry until you smell the spicy aromas from the dried red chilies. Add in the shrimp and roasted peanuts and keep stirring.

- When the shrimp are almost cooked, add the Kung Pao sauce into the wok, keep stirring until the sauce thickens. Add the chopped scallions, do a few quick stirs, dish out and serve hot.

Nutrition Facts

- Amount Per Serving (2 people)
- Calories 457
- Total Fat 26g 40%
- Saturated Fat 13g 65%
- Cholesterol 179mg 60%
- Sodium 2219mg 92%
- Potassium 509mg 15%
- Total Carbohydrates 31g 10%
- Dietary Fiber 4g 16%
- Sugars 17g
- Protein 28g 56%

- Vitamin A 24.1%
- Vitamin C 35.3%
- Calcium 10.8%
- Iron 10.4%

CREAMY THAI COCONUT CHICKEN SOUP RECIPE

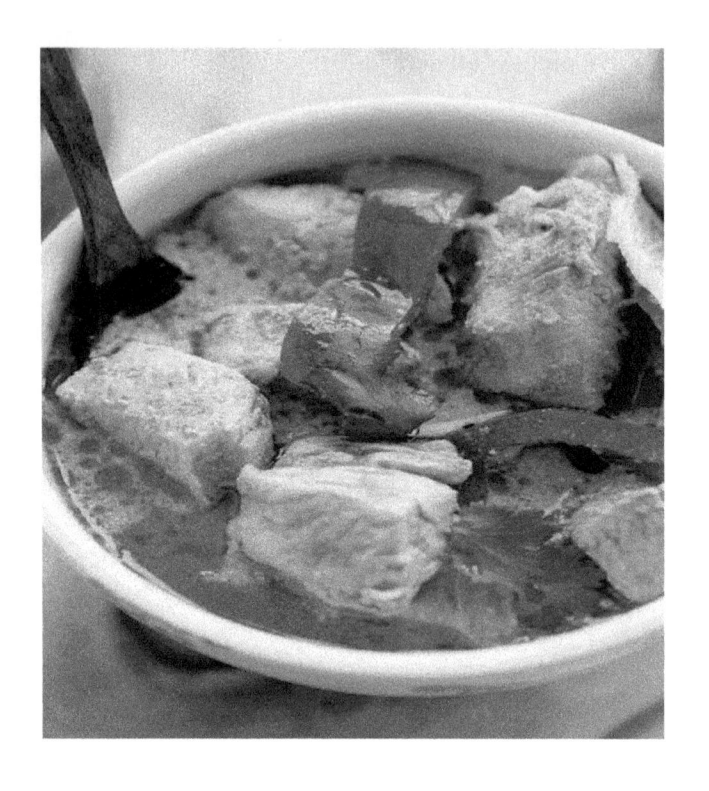

Creamy Thai Coconut Chicken Soup - easiest and fastest Thai coconut chicken recipe ever! Takes only 15 mins and dinner is ready!

Prep Time 5 minutes
Cook Time 6 minutes

Total Time 11 minutes
Servings 4 people
Calories 395 kcal

Ingredients

1. 2 tablespoons oil
2. 1 small onion, quartered
3. 2 lbs skinless and boneless chicken breast or chicken thighs, cut into cubes
4. 2 tablespoons Thai red curry paste, Mae Ploy brand
5. 1 red bell pepper, cut into thick strips
6. 6 slices galangal, optional
7. 6 kaffir lime leaves, torn and bruised, optional
8. 3 cups chicken broth
9. 2 tablespoons fish sauce or salt to taste
10. 1 tablespoon sugar
11. 3/4 cup coconut milk

12. 2 1/2 tablespoons lime juice

13. Cilantro leaves

Instructions

- Turn on the Saute mode on your Instant Pot. Add the onion and saute for 10 seconds before adding the chicken. Saute the chicken until the surface turns white. Add the Thai curry paste, bell peppers, galangal and kaffir lime leaves (if using), stir to mix well. Add the chicken broth, fish sauce and sugar. Cover the pot and select High pressure for 6 minutes.

- When it beeps, turn to Quick Release. When the valve drops, remove the lid carefully, add the coconut milk and lime juice to the soup, stir to mix well. Top with cilantro and serve immediately.

Recipe Notes

- If you can't find galangal and kaffir lime leaves (they are hard to find unless you go to a good Asian store), you can use lemongrass and skip the two ingredients. Lemongrass is not a substitute for both galangal and kaffir lime leaves but it will infuse the soup with its unique fragrance and aroma. If you don't have an Instant Pot, you can add all ingredients in the slow cooker (except coconut milk, lime juice and cilantro) and slow cook for 4-6 hours. Add the coconut milk, lime juice and cilantro when it's done cooking. You may also cook the soup on a stove. The steps are the same, except that you use a regular soup pot to cook. You may want to slowly simmer the chicken soup for about 15-20 minutes before you add the coconut milk, lime juice and cilantro.

Nutrition Facts

- Amount Per Serving (4 people)
- Calories 395
- Total Fat 22g 34%
- Saturated Fat 15g 75%
- Cholesterol 145mg 48%
- Sodium 1622mg 68%
- Potassium 1213mg 35%
- Total Carbohydrates 8g 3%
- Dietary Fiber 1g 4%
- Sugars 3g
- Protein 50g 100%
- VitaminA 43.6%
- Calcium 5%
- Iron 16.9%
- Vitamin C 71.5%

ROASTED BOK CHOY

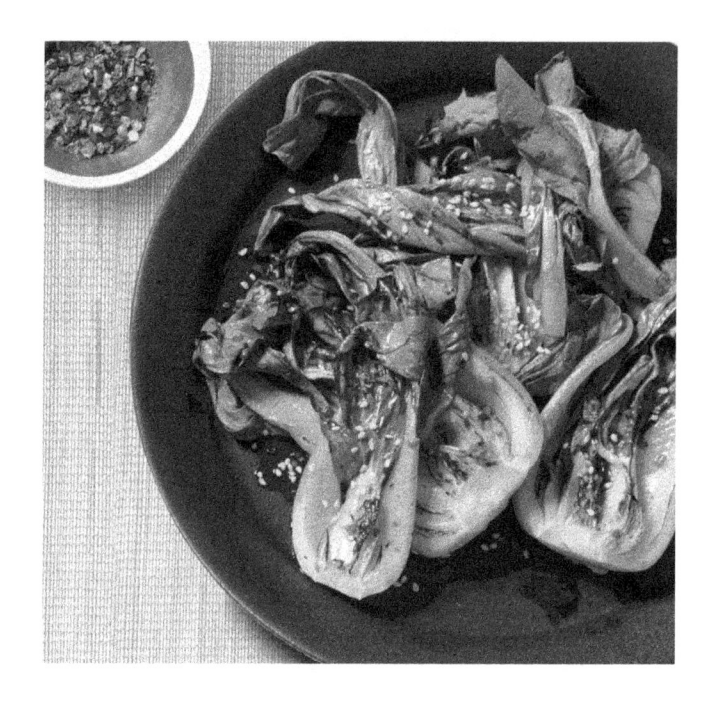

Roasted Bok Choy with Soy-Sesame sauce - learn how to roast bok choy in oven by following this easy vegetable recipe that takes only 10 mins from start to dinner. So healthy and delicious!

Prep Time 2 minutes
Cook Time 8 minutes
Total Time 10 minutes

Servings 3 people
Calories 84 kcal

Ingredients

1. 1 lb bok choy
2. 1 tablespoon olive oil
3. 3 dashes ground black pepper
4. 2 tablespoons soy sauce
5. 3/4 tablespoon sugar
6. 1/2 tablespoon apple cider vinegar
7. 1/2 teaspoon sesame oil
8. 1/4 teaspoon white sesame seeds

Instructions

- Preheat oven to 400F.
- Clean and rinse the bok choy, trim off the stems at the bottom, slice and quartered. Prepare the dressing by combining the soy

sauce, sugar, apple cider vinegar, sesame oil and sesame seeds. Stir to mix well, set aside.

- Toss the bok choy with the olive oil and black pepper. Arrange them on a baking sheet lined with parchment paper. Cover the bok choy with aluminum foil to avoid the leafy leaves from burning. You may also turn the bok choy with the inside stems down to prevent burnt leaves.

- Roast in oven for 8 minutes. Transfer the bok choy to a serving platter, drizzle the sauce and serve immediately.

Nutrition Facts

- Amount Per Serving (3 people)
- Calories 84
- Fat 51
- Total Fat 5.7g 9%
- Saturated Fat 0.8g 4%

- Sodium 700mg 29%
- Total Carbohydrates 7.2g 2%
- Dietary Fiber 1.6g 6%
- Sugars 5g
- Protein 3g 6%

BLACK PEPPER SHRIMP RECIPE

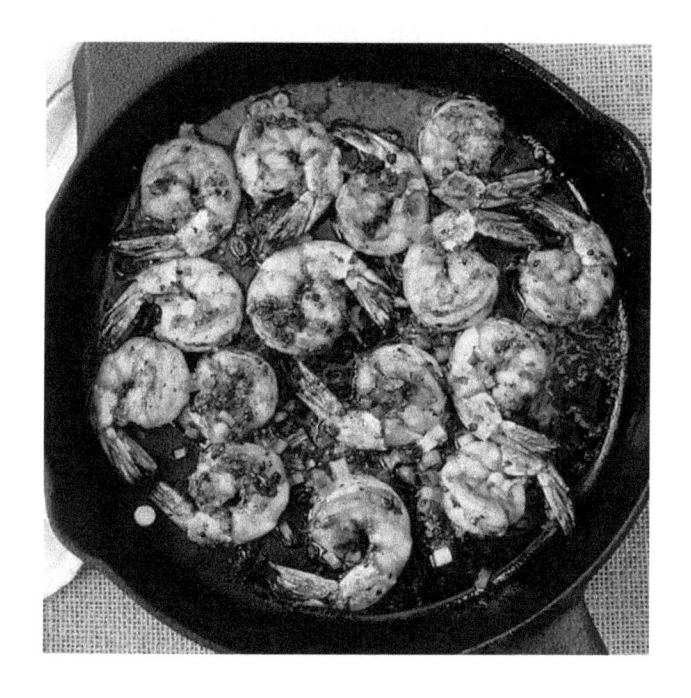

Black pepper shrimp – garlicky and buttery shrimp in a savory black pepper sauce. An easy recipe that takes 20 minutes, so delicious!

Prep Time 10 minutes
Cook Time 10 minutes
Total Time 20 minutes
Servings 3 people
Calories 198 kcal

Ingredients

1. 12 oz shell-on, headless tiger prawn or shrimp
2. 1 teaspoon black peppercorn
3. 3 tablespoon melted butter
4. 2 cloves garlic, minced
5. 1/2 tablespoon oyster sauce
6. 1 tablespoon Chinese rice wine
7. 1 teaspooon sugar
8. 1 pinch salt
9. 1 tablespoon chopped scallion

Instructions

- Remove shells from the tiger prawn or shrimp, but keep the tail on. Lightly pound the black peppercorns using a mortal and pestle until they are coarsely cracked. You may use the flat side of your knife to press, crack, and coarsely chopped the peppercorns.

- Heat up a skillet or wok and add the melted butter on medium heat. Saute the garlic and black pepper until you smell the aroma of the pepper, add the tiger prawn or shrimp and stir to combine. Add the oyster sauce, stir a few times before adding the wine and sugar. Stir fry until the prawn or shrimp are cooked. Add the scallions, stir to mix well, dish out and serve immediately.

Recipe Notes

- For the best results, broil the black pepper shrimp in the oven for 1 minute to slightly char the surface.

Nutrition Facts

- Amount Per Serving (3 people)
- Calories 198

- Total Fat 13g 20%
- Saturated Fat 7g 35%
- Cholesterol 173mg 58%
- Sodium 739mg 31%
- Potassium 148mg 4%
- Total Carbohydrates 4g 1%
- Dietary Fiber 1g 4%
- Sugars 1g
- Protein 16g 32%
- Vitamin A 11.5%
- Vitamin C 1.2%
- Calcium 7.5%
- Iron 2.1%